MORE EXERCISES IN
FETAL MONITORING

MORE EXERCISES IN FETAL MONITORING

BARRY S. SCHIFRIN, M.D.

Director
Department of Maternal-Fetal Medicine
AMI Tarzana Regional Medical Center
Tarzana, California

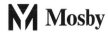 Mosby

St. Louis Baltimore Boston Chicago London Philadelphia Sydney Toronto

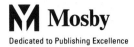

Editor: Stephanie Manning
Assistant Editor: Laura DeYoung
Project Supervisor, Production: Carol A. Reynolds
Project Supervisor, Editing: George Mary Gardner
Proofroom Manager: Barbara M. Kelly

Mosby-Year Book, Inc.
11830 Westline Industrial Drive
St. Louis, MO 63146

1 2 3 4 5 6 7 8 9 0 CL/KP 97 96 95 94 93

Library of Congress Cataloging-in-Publication Data
Schifrin, Barry S., 1938-
    More exercises in fetal monitoring / Barry S. Schifrin.
      p. cm.
    Includes bibliographical references and index.
    ISBN 0-8151-7566-3
    1. Fetal heart rate monitoring—Problems, exercises, etc.
  I. Title.
    [DNLM: 1. Fetal Monitoring—problems. 2. Heart Rate, Fetal—
problems. WQ 18 S333ml]
RG628.3.H42S35 1992
618.3′2—dc20
DNLM/DLC
for Library of Congress   92-48206
                                              CIP

To My Family

Preface

The widespread use of electronic fetal monitoring (EFM) and ultrasound for fetal surveillance has enhanced our understanding of fetal physiology and anatomy. These techniques have facilitated considerably our ability to diagnose potential abnormalities and at the same time have enhanced confidence in the diagnosis of normalcy. They have also permitted a better understanding of the limitations of the designations of "high-risk" and "low risk" pregnancy. In the ensuing material, I attempt to illustrate the problems of determining whether a pregnancy is at high or low risk. Indeed, I even classify as high risk those patients who are specifically called "low risk." The reader may not wish to indulge in this seeming persiflage, but my meaning should be clear. I believe we cannot meaningfully classify obstetrical patients as at high or low risk without incorporating fetal testing both before and during labor into the risk calculus. As many of the following tracings and commentaries suggest, too many low risk patients become high risk during labor. Low-risk and high-risk patients contribute almost equally to the census of neonatal intensive care units.

Anticipation, prevention, and timely intervention in the distressed fetus are the premise of fetal surveillance, but that is not what such monitoring does best. It best provides reassurance that fetal milestones of growth/maturity, oxygen availability, and neurologic function have been reached and that no intervention is necessary on behalf of the fetus. Pertinently, no single test, antepartum or intrapartum, informs us about all these parameters. The most popular antepartum tests are the Nonstress Test (NST) and the Biophysical Profile (BPP). The waning popularity of the contraction stress test (CST) parallels the evolving emphasis in fetal heart rate (FHR) pattern interpretation on the organization and types of responses to such intrinsic provocations as uterine contractions and fetal movement and such extrinsic provocations as vibroacoustic stimulation and maternal ingestion of food.

Fetal behavior receives only nominal attention in fetal monitoring textbooks, lectures, and workshops, where far more time is spent on decelerations, variability and the diagnosis and treatment of fetal distress. This emphasis on decelerations and variability and the search for hypoxia has resulted in a set of arbitrary guidelines for intervention and compromised the acceptance of electronic fetal monitoring. But the fetal condition cannot be truly appreciated by a "phenomenologic" approach to FHR patterns where conclusions are reached from an assessment of the number of accelerations, the type of decelerations, or the amount of variability. The term fetus, with its full complement of autonomic tone, is capable of producing a seemingly bewildering array of epochal heart rate patterns, including decelerations, which defy ready interpretation using a syntax that tends to view decreased variability as hypoxia and decelerations as a "step on the road to death." I believe we must stop focusing so narrowly on hypoxia and better appreciate the insights into fetal behavior as well as hypoxia that current surveillance permits. This book, the second in the series, is mostly about fetal behavior and its impact on FHR patterns during both antepartum and intrapartum testing.

This focus on fetal behavior does not attempt to minimize the potential significance of fetal hypoxia or its relationship to FHR patterns. Fetal asphyxia is a biochemical diagnosis with increased Pco^2 and base deficit and decreased Pco_2 and pH. Similarly, I believe that those definitions of fetal distress or fetal hypoxia that require significant neonatal distress and handicap as part of the definition should be abandoned.

FHR patterns during labor will not fail to reveal *any* significant hypoxia from any source. Depending on the source and the rapidity, the previously normal fetus responds to hypoxia first with specific decelerations (late, variable, or prolonged), and then (unless the deceleration is sustained) a rise in baseline heart rate and loss of variability before it recovers. In the absence of these usually transient changes in baseline rate, decelerations should not be considered asphyxial. The fetus that demonstrates either prolonged deceleration without recovery or progresses to a high baseline rate and decreased variability with persistent decelerations is likely undergoing significant hypoxia and may ultimately be injured or die. But whether it is actually injured at the time will, alas, take some time to tell. The FHR patterns observed during acute hypoxia should be used to "predict" subsequent neurologic handicap. As a principle, injury must be separated from asphyxia. Simply stated, one cannot determine neurologic handicap in the presence of asphyxia any more than one would be confident in predicting subsequent neurologic integrity of a person being rescued from near-drowning. I am unaware of any published evidence that suggests that a briefly asphyxiated fetus who has recovered to its previously normal baseline rate and variability within a short period of time sustains injury during that episode.

In addition to responding to asphyxial provocations, the fetus is capable of producing discernible, epochal patterns of sleep (rest), wakefulness (activity), breathing, sucking, mouthing movements, and provides in these responses insight into its neurologic functioning and maturity. In the very premature fetus there is little to distinguish these episodes. Because of the relatively high baseline rate and limited autonomic tone and maturity of the premature fetus, behavioral patterns at this stage of gestation are far more chaotic and less well organized, and the deviations in heart rate they produce less dramatic than in the older fetus. As the fetus matures, first accelerations appear, then rest-activity cycles;

and as term approaches, behavioral patterns become more complex but more obvious. In this book the words "fetal behavior" refer to recurring FHR patterns seen on the monitor strip. During labor this is synonymous with the predictable waxing and waning of variability, accelerations, and even decelerations that appear despite the stress of uterine contractions.

To take advantage of our increasing understanding of fetal behavior patterns, I have redefined the reactive NST to include analysis beyond the frequency and amplitude of accelerations. As redefined, the reactive NST not only permits the conclusion about fetal well-being (absence of asphyxia, unstressed) but normal neurologic behavior as well. This does not exclude gross abnormalities of the central nervous system. I emphasize that the reactive NST pattern cannot be counterfeited. I have also added an intermediate test result to the NST. As the fetus deteriorates, it is variability, not accelerations, that are lost first. Movements and accelerations become isolated, variability diminishes, and the sleep phase of the sleep-wake cycles is prolonged until accelerations disappears. This represents *fetal malaise,* an effect of medication, immaturity, anomaly or deterioration.

What is abnormal behavior? And how does one anticipate neurologic deficit? Abnormal behavior is most readily estimated by the *persistent* lack of variability, and is even better appreciated by studying the fetus on real-time ultrasound. Abnormal behavior may develop as a result of genetic abnormalities, malformations, as well as medication or drugs, alcohol, or a deteriorating biochemical environment; occasionally hypoxia plays a role. It appears that most fetuses who are destined to develop neurologic handicap do not show abnormal FHR patterns. As will be seen in some of the tracings, fetal anomaly or injury sometimes produces unique or bizarre FHR patterns. All aspects of the tracing may be affected, including the behavioral pattern, the baseline rate and variability, and the pattern of accelerations and decelerations. It may be that prenatal or intrapartum FHR patterns may be the most reliable determinant of subsequent neurologic outcome. In most cases, when this pattern is discovered in labor, little can be done to change the outcome. In this respect FHR patterns before and during labor may provide insight into the timing of neurologic injury. On the other hand, observation of FHR patterns during labor may provide clues to the potential development of injury. But these potential benefits and insights of monitoring are secondary. The primary role of monitoring is, again, the reassurance that all is well with the fetus. With such reassurance, administration of oxytocin or epidural anesthesia and the timing of delivery is made safer thereby.

In the outline I refer to "placental insufficiency" in two defined senses. *Respiratory insufficiency* refers to compromise of the fetal oxygen supply, a potential development at any time, but more common during labor. *Nutritional insufficiency* refers to the inability to provide adequate nourishment to the fetus, and is manifested as diminished growth, and in some instances as diminished amniotic fluid volume.

Amniotic fluid volume has been incorporated into the biophysical profile (BPP) and our preferred scheme of antepartum testing as a measure of *nutritional placental function,* not diminution in oxygen availability. Diminished amniotic fluid volume, unrelated to an anomaly or ruptured membranes, develops as part of a generalized depletion of water from the fetal compartment: from the skin, the cord, the blood volume. It does not usually represent fetal hypoxia or deterioration in *respiratory placental function.* Nutritional and respiratory deficiencies of the placenta need not develop simultaneously. It may seem paradoxical that the fetus may not flourish nutritionally despite adequate oxygenation. The clinical model here is the postmature infant, who, through dysmature, usually shows no respiratory placental insufficiency in the form of late decelerations.

Antepartum or intrapartum, test results based of FHR patterns show a relatively high false positive rate but low false negative rates. Such results have given rise to the well-known aphorism in perinatal medicine that "it is easy to make a good baby look bad, but difficult to make a bad baby look good." As a result there are numerous arguments in the literature over which test or which sequence or which criteria are "best." But which management strategy and which testing scheme is superior remains unresolved because no controlled studies have yet compared the various tests. Differences in methods, test criteria, and intervention strategy make comparisons of published data less than ideal. I believe that *testing is more important than the specific test used.* The more criteria used to define abnormality and the more often testing is carried out, the better the results. Testing also changes risk status in that the outcome of tested high-risk patients is better than that of untested, low-risk patients.

For its obvious but disputed benefits, electronic fetal monitoring cannot reliably predict outcome of problems unrelated to oxygen deprivation or those in which behavior is unaffected. Thus intrauterine growth retardation and congenital anomaly (even of the brain) usually escape detection on electronic fetal monitoring. Many hydrocephalic fetuses and even an occasional anencephalic fetus may produce seemingly normal behavioral patterns. On the other hand, there are compelling relationships between abnormal FHR patterns and the subsequent development of cerebral palsy and other forms of neurologic handicap.

The issue of routine testing has usually been deliberated as the value of the research for abnormality. This seems the wrong perspective. In an era when electronic fetal monitoring is thought to be "equivalent" to auscultation, the broadening inclusion of fetal behavior patterns into the analytic scheme seems almost anachronistic. Further, it seems, well, awkward, to continue to espouse "routine" electronic fetal monitoring both before and during labor. Testing of the individual fetus is necessary, especially during labor, to define its risk status, and may be viewed as the "well-fetus" examination. In advocating routine intrapartum monitoring I do not advocate the attachment of this "tube anchor" to the patient for the duration of her labor. Rather, I advocate, along with many others, the use of electronic fetal monitoring as an admission test when the patient first arrives. If the fetus satisfies the criteria of well-being, the monitor may be removed, to be replaced under specific situations.

I present the ensuing outlines and tracings to facilitate the understanding of FHR patterns both before and during labor. I plead guilty to minimizing the distinctions between antepartum and intrapartum FHR patterns. While it was once believed that sleep-wake cycles and fetal breathing were diminished in labor, more recent studies reveal that the fetus does cycle during early labor.

Further, I encourage the reader to assess all aspects of the tracings and appraise not only the presence or absence of fetal hypoxia but also estimate such features as gestational age and fetal responsiveness (behavior) from the clues available. The reader should formulate an opinion before reading about the outcome or considering my interpretation of the tracing. This approach attempts to maintain the uncertainty of outcome that is always present in clinical medicine. FHR tracings do not always permit accurate prediction of outcome, but they always yield the opportunity for intelligent analysis, and even reasoned disagreement.

Finally, I dare to hope that these discussions will diminish the dread of medicolegal encounters involving the allegation that a fetus was negligently injured from "perinatal asphyxia." I expect the reader to take away the following messages: That a fetus is injured does mean that it was asphyziated. That a fetus is asphyxiated does not mean that it was injured. That a fetus is injured from asphyxia does not mean that it was reasonably preventable. A reasonable management scheme is based on one of several reasonable options and takes reasonable advantage of all of the clinical information, including the FHR tracing. Such an approach, properly documented, will satisfy the most demanding standard of care, irrespective of the outcome.

Barry S. Schifrin

Contents

INTRODUCTION

HIGH-RISK PREGNANCY

DEFINITION

Pregnancy with an increased risk of poor outcome.
Alternatively, a definable segment of the population which accounts for a disproportionate share of the poor outcome.

DESIDERATA

Numbers must be manageable.
Must define risk early enough to provide therapy.
Therapy must be available.
"Low-risk" must equal negligible risk.
Contemporary medicine has not fulfilled these desiderata.
The problem lies with the "low risk" not the "high risk."

MEDICAL DISORDERS

Hypertension
Diabetes mellitus
Heart disease
Renal disease

OBSTETRICAL DISORDERS

Labor complications
Erythroblastosis
Abruptio placentae
Preeclampsia
Genital tract anomalies
Hemorrhage
Trauma
Infection

SOCIAL/DEMOGRAPHIC FACTORS

Age, parity, race
Marital status, nutrition, child spacing
Socioeconomic class, emotional factors
"Low-risk pregnancy"

COMMENTS ON HIGH-RISK STATISTICS (Table 1)

A. Less than 50% of the population remained **low-risk** throughout pregnancy.

TABLE 1.
High-Risk Statistics*

Risk Status†	Patients, No. (%)	Mortality, No./1000	Morbidity, No. (%)	DQ Mean, 1 yr
Low/low	340 (46)	1/3	22 (6.5)	106
High/low	135 (18)	3/22	16 (11.8)	105
Low/high	144 (20)	5/35	35 (24.3)	88
High/high	119 (16)	16/145	42 (35.0)	91

*From Hobel et al: 1976. Used by permission.
†Prenatal/intrapartal.
DQ = developmental quotient.

B. Thirty percent of patients initially classified **low-risk** antepartum became **high-risk** during labor.
C. Intrapartum **high-risk** carries the greatest jeopardy: intrapartum **low-risk** carries the least.
D. Antepartum low-risk patients account for about 50% of intrapartum **high risk** and poor outcome.
E. In certain centers specialized care to specific **"high-risk"** gravidas has produced outcomes comparable or better than **"low risk."**
   1. Benefit of specific care.
   2. Poverty of definition of "low risk."
F. A semantical paradox:
   1. "Low risk" = gravidas called "high risk."
   2. "High risk" = gravidas called "low risk."
   3. "Lowest risk" = gravidas receiving "optimal care."
G. Gravidas who receive no care are at highest risk.
H. Is any pregnancy **"low risk"?**

LIMITATIONS OF AVAILABLE CRITERIA

A. Clinical estimation of fetal weight:
   1. Grossly inaccurate—examiner bias.
   2. About 50% of twins not anticipated.
   3. About 50% of babies with intrauterine growth retardation (IUGR) not anticipated.
   4. Accuracy of prediction of IUGR only about 50%.
   5. Accuracy unrelated to experience.
B. Ultrasound estimation of fetal weight:
   1. Better than clinical estimation.
   2. Average error about 10%.
   3. Error greater at extremes of birth weight.
C. The "weighting game":
   1. The accuracy of estimating fetal weight lies not with how closely you predict the fetal weight, but how well you assign the patient to a proper management scheme.

2. As the estimated birth weight at which we are prepared to intervene for fetal benefit decreases, it is only necessary to decide whether the fetus is too small to profit from aggressive care.
3. An example: Assume that you are prepared to intervene, on indication, in a fetus whose estimated birth weight is 650 g. If the fetus weighs 675 g but your estimate is 635 g and you do not intervene because the fetus is "too small," you have assigned the fetus to the wrong management strategy—despite an error of 40 g (or 6%).
4. There are only two questions to be answered:
   Is the fetus too young to profit from enlightened care?
   Is the fetus too large to deliver from below?

D. Clinical auscultation of the fetal heart:
1. Intermittent.
2. Errors introduced: technique, listener bias.
3. Detection of fetal distress depends on:
   a. Rate signifying distress: 120, 100, 80 bpm.
   b. Fetal baseline heart rate
   c. Detection of contractions
   d. Duration and amplitude of decelerations
   e. Onset and duration of counting
4. Cannot assess variability.
5. Confined to period between contractions.
6. Does not predict early distress during labor or before.
7. Does not predict deterioration or mechanism of distress.
8. Experience unrelated to accuracy.
9. Unrelated to outcome.
10. Randomized controlled trials show no benefit of auscultation in prediction of fetal condition irrespective of attention or scheme.
11. Cannot reproduce fetal heart rate (FHR) patterns from auscultation (Miller et al.).
12. Clinically unrealistic.
13. Impractical; too expensive to provide sufficient nursing.

TO IMPROVE STATISTICS

A. Understand limitations of available methods of fetal evaluation.
B. Risk status of the fetus must be tested directly before assigning any mother to "low-risk status."

ELEMENTS OF FETAL SURVEILLANCE

A. Growth/nutrition:
1. Sequential ultrasonic mensuration:
   a. Biparietal diameter (BPD), femur length, abdominal circumference.
   b. Head/abdomen ratio.
   c. Bowel pattern, epiphyses, etc.

2. Amniotic fluid volume (AFV):
   a. Diminution in AFV with IUGR not related to hypoxia.
   b. No chronic hypoxic model produces oligohydramnios.
B. Oxygenation:
1. pH, blood gases—experimental percutaneous umbilical blood sampling (PUBS)
2. Contraction stress test [CST] and breast stimulation test [BST])
C. Neurological integrity—behavior:
1. Non-stress test (NST).
2. Biophysical profile.
D. Placental insufficiency:
1. Poorly defined term, as a minimum:
   a. **Respiratory placental insufficiency**
      (1) Transport of oxygen, gases, maintenance of pH.
      (2) Requires ongoing maintenance at high level.
   b. **Nutritional placental insufficiency:**
      (1) Transport of nutrients.
      (2) May be curtailed transiently without embarrassment.
   c. Paradox: May have interference of nutritional function without impairment of respiratory function, e.g. postdate
E. Questions, questions, questions
1. Questions *to ask yourself* before you test:
   a. What am I testing for?
   b. Can the information be obtained clinically?
   c. Can an abnormality be predicted specifically?
   d. What is the risk of the procedure?
   e. Can a clinical decision be based on the result?
   f. Are we monitoring the inevitable?
   g. Is the test simple, safe, rapid?
   h. Is the stress tolerable, transient, quantifiable?
   i. Is the end point measurable, reproducible, sensitive?
   j. Does the end point depend on gestational age?
   k. How much does it cost?
   l. Do I have a plan for each possible result?
2. Questions *not to ask the fetus:*
   a. How old are you?
   b. How much do you weigh?
   c. What's your lecithin-sphingomyelin (L/S) ratio?
   d. Do you have any decelerations?
3. Questions *to ask the fetus:*
   a. How are you doing in there?
   b. Are you behaving yourself properly?
   c. Is there something your mother can do?
   d. Would you prefer to be somewhere else?
   e. Do you have a burning desire to meet a pediatrician?

f. Are you too large for safe vaginal delivery?

g. Are you too premature to benefit from modern care?

NON-STRESS TEST

A. Technique for assessing fetal well-being by observing the fetal heart rate (FHR) response to spontaneous or induced fetal movement (FM). Includes epochal responses (rest-activity cycles).

B. Reactive pattern suggests:
 1. Normal neurological control.
 2. Adequate oxygenation (unstressed).

C. NST does not define:
 1. Nutritional growth failure.
 2. Anomalies.

CONTRACTION STRESS TEST

A. Technique for assessing fetoplacental respiratory reserve by observing the fetal heart rate (FHR) response to spontaneous or induced uterine contractions (UC).

B. Negative CST precludes hypoxia.

C. CST does not define:
 1. Nutritional growth failure.
 2. Anomalies.
 3. Pre-existing neurological injury.

BIOPHYSICAL PROFILE (BPP)

A. Technique for assessing fetal well-being by observing responses of fetal heart rate to fetal movement (NST), fetal body movement (FM), fetal breathing movements (FBM), fetal tone (TON), and quantifying amniotic fluid volume (AFV).

B. Placental grade included in some schemes.

C. Permits a general survey of intrauterine contents including presentation, position, BPD, placental localization, IUGR, anomalies.

D. Normal test suggests:
 1. Normal neurological control.
 2. Adequate oxygenation (unstressed).
 3. Nutritional adequacy.

INDICATIONS FOR TESTING

A. Patients at increased risk for placental insufficiency, e.g., diabetes, toxemia, hypertension, postdate.

B. When other examinations suggest fetal compromise:
 1. Suspect IUGR, oligohydramnios, multiple gestation.
 2. Meconium staining of amniotic fluid, etc.

C. When events or complaints dictate:
 1. Decreased fetal movement.
 2. Trauma, bloody amniocentesis.

D. Routine antepartum surveillance.

CONTRAINDICATIONS TO TESTING

A. NST/profile—none.

B. Contraindications to induction of contractions:
 1. Vaginal bleeding.
 2. Ruptured membranes.
 3. Previous cesarean section.
 4. Polyhydramnios.
 5. Multiple gestation.
 6. Incompetent cervix.
 7. Other contraindications to labor.

TESTING PROCEDURES

A. Patients should refrain from smoking; test after meals; position: semi-Fowler's, left lateral-tilt, avoid supine.

B. Carry out testing in a quiet room, free from distractions; take BP every 10 to 15 minutes; obtain first BP in either sitting or lateral position.

C. Position external FHR transducer for best recording.

D. Position external tocotransducer over the uterine fundus or fetal trunk or extremity (to record breathing movements).

E. Determine baseline FHR, variability, accelerations, decelerations, fetal movements, and uterine contractions.

F. Record name, date, time of day, medication, indication, vital signs, position, monitoring technique, etc.

G. If NST nonreactive after 20 minutes stimulate fetus:
 1. Abdominal palpation.
 2. Glucose-containing beverage to mother.
 3. Vibroacoustic stimulus (see below).

H. Vibroacoustic stimulation.
 1. Apparatus
  a. Electronic larynx (Western Electric)
  b. Acoustic stimulator
 2. Technique
  a. Apply to region of fetal head
  b. Single, short buzz

I. For CST, induce uterine contractions if:
 1. Spontaneous UC less than 3/10 minutes.
 2. No repeated late decelerations.

3. Nonreactive NST.
4. You are hoping to induce labor.
J. Oxytocin infusion:
   1. Administer by constant infusion pump.
   2. Initial rate—0.5 to 1.0 mU/minute.
   3. Increase rate by 1 mU/minute every 15 to 30 minutes until there are three UCs lasting 40 seconds in 10-minute window.
   4. Starting dosage and rate of oxytocin increase empirical; may need to start slower to avoid hypertonus.
K. Breast stimulation:
   1. Ensure privacy.
   2. Numerous variations on technique:
      a. Unilateral—bilateral.
      b. Exposed—unexposed.
      c. Warm towel—fingers only.
      d. Continuous—intermittent.
      e. Nipple roll—palpation—breast pump.
   3. Minimum frequency of hypertonus with intermittent, unilateral palpation.
L. Discontinue oxytocin infusion or breast stimulation if:
   1. Satisfactory test (positive or negative CST).
   2. Unsatisfactory data.
   3. Equivocal CST despite 1 hour of satisfactory UCs.
   4. Infusion rate greater than 16 mU/minute (arbitrary); sometimes higher infusion rates necessary.
   5. After 15 minutes of breast stimulation.
   6. If contractions are:
      a. Less than 2 minutes apart or more frequently than three in 10 minutes.
      b. Last longer than 60 seconds.
   7. Prolonged fetal deceleration.
M. Response to hypertonus:
   1. Discontinue oxytocin or breast stimulation.
   2. Lateral position.
   3. Oxygen by face mask.
   4. Check maternal vital signs.
   5. Uterine relaxant (e.g., terbutaline).
N. Continue to monitor until contractions return to baseline level.
O. Irrespective of designation of test or stimulus applied (NST, CST, BST) evaluate for:
   1. Movements and fetal responses thereto.
   2. Contractions and fetal responses thereto.
P. BPP—perform general survey of intrauterine contents, including: presentation, position, biparietal diameter, placental localization; during this survey and for 10 to 30 minutes thereafter, FM, FBM are counted and TON determined.

Q. Monitoring twins:
   1. Must monitor twins simultaneously.
   2. Procedure facilitated by preliminary ultrasound.
   3. If using two monitors, mark tracings simultaneously.
R. Documentation:
   1. Record interpretation—and criteria.
   2. Obtain official reading (if required).
   3. Obtain consultation (if required).
   4. Disposition—home, hospital, office, etc.
   5. Save tracing—original, microfilm, or laser storage.
   6. Annotate stimulation, etc.

COMPLICATIONS OF TESTING

A. CST:
   1. Hypertonus, fetal distress.
   2. Preterm labor (theoretical).
B. Vibroacoustic stimulation—all theoretical:
   1. Produces sound and vibration:
      a. Represents energy input into uterus.
      b. Sound in utero may be louder than in air.
      c. Effects related to intensity, duration, and frequency of stimulation.
   2. Mechanism of response may involve pain in fetus with release of catecholamines—disputed.
   3. Generally regarded as safe:
      a. Apparently normal auditory function in babies
      b. Should probably avoid with oligohydramnios.
C. All: misinterpretation of results.

TIMING AND FREQUENCY OF TESTING

A. Begin testing at time when results will be acted on.
B. "Low risk"—at 32 to 34, 38, and 40 weeks (arbitrary).
C. "High risk":
   1. Weekly, except:
      a. Semi-weekly:
         (1) Risk of oligohydramnios (IUGR, postdates).
         (2) Diabetes mellitus.
   2. Daily: certain preterm premature rupture of membranes (PROM) unstable conditions.
D. No testing interval guarantees normal outcome.

RESPONSE TO ANTEPARTUM TESTS

A. Normal test results:
   1. No fetal indication for intervention.
   2. Repeat as clinically indicated.
B. Abnormal test results:
   1. Continue monitoring.

2. Repeat test according to plan.
3. Induction of labor.
4. Cesarean section.

C. Documentation of thought process.

CLASSIFICATION OF RESULTS

NON-STRESS TEST

REACTIVE NON-STRESS TEST (NST-R)

Acceleration amplitude: At least 15 bpm from baseline to peak; before 32 weeks, use 10 bpm for 15 seconds.

Acceleration duration: At least 15 seconds from onset to return.

Acceleration frequency: Two or more FHR accelerations in 10 minutes. At least 2 accelerations must coalesce.

Variability: Average sleep-wake cycles.

Note: Auscultated accelerations acceptable.

NONREACTIVE NON-STRESS TEST (NST-NR)

Acceleration amplitude: Less than 15 bpm from baseline to peak.

Acceleration duration: Less than 15 seconds from onset to return, *or*

Acceleration frequency: Less than 2 in 10 minutes, *or* accelerations do not coalesce.

Variability: Persistently decreased.

Note: If intermediate classification used then NST-NR refers to: absent accelerations *and* decreased variability.

INTERMEDIATE NON-STRESS TEST (NST-I)

Acceleration amplitude: At least 15 bpm from baseline to peak.

Acceleration duration: At least 15 seconds from onset to return.

Acceleration frequency: At least 1 in 10 minutes; accelerations do not coalesce.

Variability: Persistently decreased.

SINUSOIDAL NON-STRESS TEST (NST-S)

Sine wave amplitude: 5 to 15 bpm (some greater).

Sine wave frequency: 3 to 6 cycles per minute (cpm).

Absent variability and reactivity; variant of NST-NR.

UNSATISFACTORY NON-STRESS TEST (NST-U)

Technically poor tracing: precludes detection of accelerations.

CONTRACTION STRESS TEST

NEGATIVE CONTRACTION STRESS TEST (CST-N)

Absent decelerations with three palpable UCs in 10 minutes.

POSITIVE CONTRACTION STRESS TEST (CST-P)

Recurrent late decelerations with three UCs in 10 minutes.

EQUIVOCAL CONTRACTION STRESS TEST (CST-E)

Inability to define either a negative or positive CST within 1 hour of satisfactory testing.

Recurrent non-late decelerations.

UNSATISFACTORY CONTRACTION STRESS TEST (CST-U)

Technically poor tracing
or
Inability to obtain three UCs in 10 minutes within 1 hour.

BIOPHYSICAL PROFILE

FETAL BREATHING MOVEMENTS PRESENT (FBM-P)

One or more episodes of fetal breathing lasting at least 60 seconds within a 10-minute period.

FETAL BREATHING MOVEMENTS ABSENT (FBM-A)

No episode of fetal breathing within 10 minutes.

FETAL BODY MOVEMENTS PRESENT (FM-P)

At least three discrete episodes of limb or trunk movements within a 10-minute period. Simultaneous movements are counted as a single movement.

FETAL BODY MOVEMENTS DECREASED (FM-D)

Fewer than three discrete FMs in 10-minute period.

FETAL MUSCLE TONE NORMAL (TON-N)

Upper and lower extremities in full flexion.
Trunk in position of flexion and head flexed on chest.
At least one episode of extension of extremities or extension of spine with return to position of flexion.

FETAL BODY MOVEMENTS DECREASED (TON-D)

Extremities extended or partially flexed.
Fetal spine extended, hand open.
Fetal movement not followed by return to flexion.

AMNIOTIC FLUID VOLUME NORMAL (AFV-N)

Fluid evident throughout uterine cavity.
Largest vertical pocket of fluid > 2 cm.
Amniotic fluid index > 10.

AMNIOTIC FLUID VOLUME DECREASED (AFV-D):

Fluid absent in most areas of uterine cavity.
Largest fluid pocket < 2.5 cm in vertical axis.
Crowding of fetal small parts.
Amniotic fluid index (AFI) < 5 cm

AMNIOTIC FLUID VOLUME INCREASED (AFV-I):

Overt polyhydramnios; largest pocket > 8 cm.

FETAL BEHAVIOR

BEHAVIOR STATES: CLASSIFICATION BY FETAL ACTIVITIES

States 1F–4F (Table 2).
Organization normally present by 36 to 38 weeks.
Generally, FBM and FM don't occur simultaneously.
State affects variables used to test fetal well-being, FBM, FM, and FHR.

AS GESTATION ADVANCES

A. Heart rate patterns:
1. Mean heart rate decreases and variability increases.
2. Cycles more obvious, accelerations more pronounced, epochal; fewer decelerations with activity.
3. Circadian rhythm:
    a. Peak between 0800 and 0900.
    b. Trough between 0100 and 0400—may reach levels down to 90 to 100 bpm.
4. Before 28 weeks, epochal changes rarely dramatic.
5. About 65% reactive at 28 weeks.
6. About 95% reactive at 34 weeks.
7. Nonreactive NST as function of prematurity applies only if there has been no previous reactive NST.

RESPONSES TO VIBROACOUSTIC STIMULATION

A. Fetal heart rate responses:
1. Tachycardia, accelerations.
2. Amplitude inversely proportional to baseline rate.
3. Responses may last 30 minutes or longer.
4. Abnormal response: bradycardia or decelerations.
B. Ultrasound responses:
1. Startle.
2. Head movements, sucking, swallowing.
3. Alteration of fetal state.
C. Responses influenced by:
1. Fetal state:
    a. State 1: most easily aroused.
    b. State 2: least responsive.
2. Duration, intensity, and frequency of stimulus.

TABLE 2.

Fetal Behavioral States

State	Baseline	Variability	Accelerations	Body Movements	Breathing Movements	Eye Movements
1—quiet sleep	Stable	Decreased	Rare	Brief, absent	Infrequent, regular	Absent
2—REM sleep	Stable	Increased	Episodic with fetal movement	Episodic, gross truncal flexion/extension	Frequent, irregular	Present
3—similar to state 1	Stable	Average	Absent	Absent	Infrequent, absent	Present
4—active sleep	Unstable tachycardia	Increased	Large	Continuous gross truncal	Present, irregular	Present

D. Vibroacoustic stimulation
  1. Before 32 weeks:
     a. No increase in accelerations, tachycardia
     b. Startle response—brief
  2. After 32 weeks:
     a. Increases number of body movements
     b. Decreases respiratory movements
     c. Habituation to response
E. Mechanisms—not proven:
  1. Vibration stimulus.
  2. Auditory pain.
  3. Catecholamine release—disputed.

EFFECTS OF DRUGS ON BEHAVIOR

A. Barbiturates, tranquilizers:
  1. Decrease the incidence of REM sleep.
  2. Prolong periods of HVECOG.
  3. Decreased variability, isolated accelerations.
B. Cocaine:
  1. Atypical, disorganized, or bizarre behavior.
  2. Disrupted behavior in response to stimulation.
  3. Sustained hyperpnea, recurrent yawning.
  4. Hypertonic and hyperirritable.
  5. May never attain organized state BEHAVIOR by term.
  6. Difficult to arouse, difficult to console.
  7. Lack of habituation.
  8. Persistently nonreactive NST.
  9. Persistently reactive NST.
  10. Mimics "all or none" or "wired" neonate.

FETAL MOVEMENTS

A. Detection:
  1. Seen by ultrasound as early as 6 to 7 weeks.
  2. Felt by patient 16 to 20 weeks (quickening).
  3. Peak activity 28 to 32 weeks, declines thereafter.
  4. Wide range of normal activity, diurnal variation.
  5. Patient detection varies (about 75%).
B. Movements become more complex, sustained as fetus matures.
C. Physiology:
  1. Occur during LVECOG and HVECOG—frequent.
  2. Abolished by hypoxia, medication, smoking, etc.
  3. Stimulated by contractions.
  4. Coincide with accelerations.
  5. Begins as early as 7.5 weeks gestation.
  6. Later stretching or rolling movements.
  7. Gross movements episodic—about 10% of time.
  8. May be absent for as long as 75 minutes.
  9. Interchangeable with FHR accelerations.

FETAL BREATHING MOVEMENTS

A. Frequently associated with rapid eye movements (REM).
B. Associated with lower rate, increased variability; sometimes regular oscillatory pattern.
C. Occasionally associated with "late decelerations" if UC present.
D. Usually not associated with fetal movements.

E. Episodic—apnea up to 120 minutes in normals; usually less.
F. During LVECOG.
G. Circadian rhythm in healthy fetuses.
H. Increased:
   1. Glucose infusion (fasting).
   2. Hypercapnea.
   3. Smoking.
   4. Prostaglandin synthetase inhibitors.
   5. Normal fetus develops tolerance.
   6. After meals and during sleep.
I. Decreased in:
   1. Hypoxemia (normocapnea).
   2. Asphyxia—gasping.
   3. Alcohol—not reversed by glucose.
J. Recognized in human as early as 10 weeks.
K. Gestation dependent:
   1. Between 24 to 28 weeks' gestation: 10% to 20%.
   2. Beyond 30 weeks' gestation: 30% to 40%.

FETAL TONE

A. Least reliable parameter and last one to go.
B. Hard to detect with decreased AFV.

AMNIOTIC FLUID VOLUME

A. Increased:
   1. Diabetes, Rh isoimmunization, hydrops fetalis (most).
   2. Anomalies—genitourinary (GU), neurologic.
   3. Miscellaneous.
B. Decreased:
   1. Ruptured membranes.
   2. Hypertensive disorders, IUGR—asymmetrical, postdate.
   3. Anomalies—GU.
   4. If prolonged—acquired pulmonary, renal, orthopedic changes.
   5. Miscellaneous.

UTERINE CONTRACTIONS

A. Composed of high-frequency, low-amplitude oscillations with occasional high-amplitude, low frequency contractions (Braxton-Hicks).
B. As gestation advances, low-amplitude oscillations disappear, UC become more frequent, eventually evolve into labor.
C. Hypertonus/tetany:
   1. Spontaneous—about 2%.
   2. Oxytocin infusion—about 5%.
   3. Breast stimulation—about 5%, depending on technique.

D. Behavioral responses to uterine contractions:
   1. Initially stimulate fetal movement.
   2. Later stimulate fetal breathing.

DECREASED VARIABILITY

A. Decelerations absent:
   1. Rest state.
   2. Medication.
   3. Late hypoxia—with unstable baseline.
   4. Neurological deficit—injury or anomaly.
B. Decelerations present—asphyxia.
C. Occasionally "sinusoidal."

INCREASED VARIABILITY

A. With frequent movements; actually reactivity.
B. With low baseline, especially postdates.
C. After variable decelerations.
D. Usually not ominous sign.

SINUSOIDAL PATTERN

A. Consider diagnosis only in the absence of reactivity anywhere.
B. Variant of decreased (short-term) variability.
C. Characteristics:
   1. Amplitude: 5 to 15 bpm.
   2. Frequency: 3 to 6 cpm.
   3. These features same as normal, with variability.
D. Mechanism:
   1. Uncertain.
   2. Possibly related to endorphin release:
      a. May be induced by narcotics.
      b. May be relieved by naloxone HCl (Narcan).
      c. Probably not vagal effect.
E. Clinical classification:
   1. Ominous pattern:
      a. Rh isoimmunization or fetal anemia.
      b. Neurologic injury; usually other features.
      c. Preceding death; other ominous features.
      d. Usually sporadic, sometimes persistent.
   2. Benign pattern:
      a. No identifiable cause.
      b. Narcotic administration.
      c. May be episodic or persistent.
   3. Congenital anomaly:
      a. Seen with cardiac, CNS anomalies.
      b. Usually persistent.

F. Intervention probably not indicated solely on basis of sinusoidal pattern.

BASELINE BRADYCARDIA

A. Definition: baseline FHR less than 110 bpm.
B. Incidence: 5% to 10% of antepartum tests—often postdate.
C. Majority associated with reactive NST.
D. At 60 to 80 bpm may represent congenital heart block, which is invariably associated with a nonreactive NST.
E. Seen occasionally with hypoglycemia, drugs (i.e., propanolol), hypothermia.
F. Bradycardia is a very late sign of fetal asphyxia. More often associated with late term or postterm fetus. Other features usually present, including:
   1. Unstable baseline rate.
   2. Absent variability.
   3. Decelerations or accelerations.
G. Not a reliable sign of fetal distress or an end point of the NST or CST.

BASELINE TACHYCARDIA

A. Definition—baseline FHR greater than 150 bpm.
B. Incidence—about 10% to 15% of antepartum tests.
C. While sicker babies tend to have higher average rates they are rarely in the tachycardia range; tachycardia is not a reliable sign of fetal distress or an end point for the NST or CST.
D. Occasionally may represent coalescence of accelerations with fetal movement in active fetus (reactive NST).
E. In sequential testing, rate remains stable or falls slightly.
   1. If rate rises—even if not > 150, consider as abnormal.
   2. In postdate baby, rate ≥ 150 bpm suggests deterioration.
F. Maternal anxiety, smoking, ketosis.
G. Medication: atropine, β-mimetics.

DECELERATIONS

A. Variable decelerations:
   1. Seen in about 10% of NST, up to 25% of CST—most common deceleration.
   2. Increased with UC; frequent with oligohydramnios.
   3. Usually seen with reactive NST; associated with FM.
   4. Variable decelerations with flat baseline and nonreactive NST may be an ominous pattern ("atypical variables" or "overshoot").
   5. Provoked with "cord maneuvers" (fundal pressure, palpation of fetal neck).
   6. In preterm fetus, may accompany normal fetal movement.

B. Late decelerations (positive CST):
   1. Uncommon, especially with reactive pattern—all false-positive CST.
   2. With hypotension or oxytocin can induce in any fetus.
   3. Usually ominous with nonreactive NST.
   4. Occasionally seen with spontaneous hypertonus.
   5. May represent fetal breathing movement—usually associated with reactive NST; no rise in FHR or loss of variability.
   6. Criteria—all must apply:
      a. Uniform, symmetrical, repetitive.
      b. Onset after onset of uterine contraction.
      c. Duration proportional to duration of UC.
      d. Amplitude proportional to amplitude of UC.
      e. In normal fetus, must induce transient rise in baseline, decrease in variability.
C. Prolonged decelerations:
   1. Uncommon, usually associated with uterine hypertonus.
   2. Oligohydramnios.
   3. In certain postdate pregnancies: Prolonged (4–6 minutes), shallow (<30 bpm) decelerations with normal variability, stable baseline. Do not confuse with late decelerations but consider for delivery.

SPORADIC ACCELERATIONS

A. Uniform, symmetrical accelerations unassociated with contractions or periodic decelerations.
B. Seen with fetal movement or stimulation:
   1. Represents integrative response of fetal CNS.
   2. Basis of reactive NST.
C. Characteristics—crucial to definition of R-NST:
   1. Arise from normal variability.
   2. Variability reduced at peak of deceleration.
   3. Somewhat irregular; slower rise, faster fall.
   4. Tend to coalesce, may appear as tachycardia (scalloped or sustained).
   5. Return may transiently undershoot baseline (lambda pattern).
   6. Appear about simultaneously with FM.
   7. Average duration: 30 to 60 seconds.
   8. Average amplitude: 20 to 25 bpm; inversely proportional to baseline rate.
   9. Mean interval: 45 to 85 seconds! (Compare to criteria of 2/10 minutes.)
   10. Occasionally exaggerated; probably benign.

UNIFORM ACCELERATIONS

A. Uniform, symmetrical.
B. Coincident with uterine contractions.
C. Reflects shape of contraction.
D. Occurrence:
   1. Early in labor—before membranes ruptured.
   2. Following atropine administration.
   3. Common in nonvertex presentations.
   4. Deterioration of NST (with absent variability).
E. Apparently benign response with normal variability.

VARIABLE ACCELERATIONS

A. More properly classified with variable decelerations.
B. Variably shaped accelerations which do not reflect shape of UC.
   1. "Shoulders" on variable decelerations.
   2. As feature of "increased variability" with contractions.
   3. Usually associated with average baseline variability.
C. Apparently benign response.

REBOUND ACCELERATIONS (OVERSHOOT)

A. More properly classified with variable decelerations.
B. Uniform accelerations following variable decelerations.
C. Characteristics—all must apply
   1. Smooth baseline—*persistently* absent variability and reactivity.
   2. Follows variable deceleration regardless of amplitude.
   3. Usual duration—longer than 12 seconds.
   4. Occasionally, acceleration more prominent than preceding deceleration.
   5. May also be seen:
      a. Following administration of atropine.
      b. Immature fetus.
      c. Excessive tachycardia of any cause.
   6. Do not confuse with exaggerated variable accelerations following moderate-severe variable decelerations.
   7. Do not confuse with occasional decelerations in otherwise reactive fetus.
D. Ominous commentary on variable deceleration.

COMMENTS ON PROCEDURES

NST

A. Attempt to find reactive window within 40 minutes. Normal sleep-wake cycles about 20 to 40 minutes. Extending test to 80 minutes yields an additional 2% reactive.
B. Reactive pattern cannot be counterfeited! Consider pattern reactive irrespective of stimulus used or time required. If stimulus used, the response must be interpreted exactly as described for spontaneous movement.
C. During sleep/rest part of cycle, variability may be absent. The older the fetus the less variability during the sleep part of the cycle.
D. Especially on early monitors, external FHR techniques tended to exaggerate variability; when such recordings indicate decreased variability, it is probably genuine.
E. Frequency of reactive pattern depends on:
   1. Gestational age, risk status.
   2. Medication: sedatives, propanolol, smoking.
   3. Criteria, duration, and conditions of testing.
   4. Normal fetus may show variability, not accelerations.
   5. Fetus with tachycardia may not show accelerations or respond to VAS.
F. Deterioration of NST:
   1. Breakup of rest-activity cycles; longer sleep cycles.
   2. Decreased variability.
   3. Isolated accelerations.
   4. Rise in baseline (variable).
   5. Loss of accelerations.
   6. Variable decelerations with overshoot.
G. Vibroacoustic stimulation
   1. Restricted usefulness with
      a. IUGR and oligohydramnios
      b. Nuchal cord
      c. During labor with ruptured membranes
   2. Choice of response:
      a. Reactivity—all criteria for R-NST.
      b. Isolated acceleration—not acceptable.
   3. Interpretation of normal response:
      a. Hypoxia—absent.
      b. Neurological integrity—intact.
      c. Hearing—intact.
   4. Caveats:
      a. Absence of a response does not necessarily indicate hypoxia or dysfunction.
      b. Appearance of accelerations does not necessarily represent state change!
      c. Response does not imply that higher cortical centers of fetus are intact.
      d. Accelerations not a comprehensive indicator of fetal well-being.
H. Reversible distress:
   1. Maternal ketoacidosis—tachycardia, decelerations.
   2. Maternal hypoglycemia—bradycardia.

3. Maternal hypothermia—bradycardia.
4. Maternal exercise—tachycardia, decelerations.
5. Maternal anxiety, stress—tachycardia.
6. External version—prolonged decelerations.
7. Maternal hypoxia—decelerations.
8. Fetal anemia—sinusoidal pattern, decelerations.
9. Fetal arrhythmia—tachycardia, heart failure.
10. Drug intake—various changes.
I. Improving resolution of nonreactive NST.
  1. Repeating test—usually after meals.
  2. Extending test up to 80 to 120 minutes.
  3. Attention to criteria—see intermediate NST.
  4. Stimulation—VAS, glucose, palpation, stress.
  5. Corroboration with other tests—CST, BPP.
J. Finally, the *non-stress test* is poorly named.

CST

A. Attempt to find positive or negative 10-minute window.
B. Only criteria for positive CST is late decelerations with UC; reactivity is not an end point of the CST.
C. With sufficient oxytocin or maternal hypotension, can induce late decelerations in any fetus. Also, may induce variable decelerations, especially with oligohydramnios (a benefit).
D. Anomalous fetuses—disproportionate share of abnormal CSTs.
E. Disadvantages:
  1. Cumbersome.
  2. Time consuming.
  3. Patient discomfort.
  4. Can't quantify stress.
  5. Infrequent positive, high false-positive rate.
  6. Poor predictors of outcome.
F. Benefits of BST vs. CST:
  1. Requires less time (45 vs. 90 minutes).
  2. Simpler.
  3. Better patient acceptance.
  4. Success rate increases with advancing gestational age.
G. Drawbacks of BST:
  1. Higher risk of hypertonus.
  2. Less successful than CST (70% vs. 95%).
  3. Increases likelihood of hypertonus with later oxytocin.

BIOPHYSICAL PROFILE

A. Consists of two classes of parameters:
  1. Dynamic/epochal (NST, FBM, FM, TON).
  2. Static (AFV).

B. Dynamic parameters all related generally:
  1. All present, though not at the same time.
  2. When fetus moving and accelerating generally not breathing.
  3. Multiple parameters do not improve definition of normal.
  4. If NST reactive other dynamic signs of no added benefit.
  5. May include eye, tongue, mouth movement.
  6. Fetus invariably affected when all parameters abnormal.
C. Diminished AFV (recent):
  1. Associated with:
    a. Meconium.
    b. Decelerations—usually variable.
    c. Dysmaturity syndrome—wasting, skin/orthopedic changes.
  2. About 40% of patients with decreased AFV have decelerations during the NST and labor.
  3. About 90% of postdate patients with decelerations during NST have decreased AFV.
  4. Intermittent umbilical cord compression probably predisposes to fetal death, neurological injury, especially if associated with IUGR, postmaturity.
  5. Occasionally, rapid diminution in AFV within 24 hours.
  6. With adequate AFV, infant rarely has postmaturity syndrome.
  7. Evolving criteria for height of vertical pocket.
  8. Prostaglandin antagonists: Aspirin and indomethacin reduce urine output, decrease AFV.

SCORING SYSTEMS

  1. BPP planning score (Platt, Manning):
    0 or 2 points for each parameter—maximum 10.
  2. BPP scoring system (Vintzeleos et al.):
    Includes placental grade:
    0, 1, 2 points for each parameter—maximum 12.
  3. NST scoring systems (Fischer, Krebs, Lyons).
  4. Implications for therapy depend on reactivity and AFV not score.
  5. Scores tend to detract from understanding.

FETAL MOVEMENT TESTING (KICK COUNTS, ETC.):

  1. Convenient, universal, inexpensive.
  2. When movements present, at least 97% show reactive NSTs.
  3. Patient participation.
  4. If patient claims decreased FM—must get NST; at least 50% of tests will be normal.

5. Some neurologically handicapped fetuses move.
6. Pitfalls—uncertainty about temporal relationship between decreased FM and fetal deterioration.
7. Emotional pitfall—making patient responsible invites her inference that she failed if fetus does poorly.
8. Mechanism:
   a. Fetal deterioration.
   b. Drug effect on fetus.
   c. Oligohydramnios.
   d. Polyhydramnios.
   e. Maternal perception problem.

FHR PATTERNS AND SUBSEQUENT NEUROLOGICAL HANDICAP

Asphyxia	Electronic Fetal Monitoring	
	Fetal behavioral patterns	
	Normal	Abnormal
Absent	**Reassuring**	**Suspicious** Drugs, prematurity, anomaly, injury
Present	**Threatening** Recoverable fetal distress	**Pathological** Uncompensated fetal distress

Asphyxia	Electronic Fetal Monitoring	
	Fetal behavioral patterns	
	Normal	Abnormal
Absent	**Reassuring** Variability present, accelerations present, rest-activity cycles	**Suspicious** Variability absent, accelerations absent, decelerations absent
Present	**Threatening** Variability present, decelerations present	**Pathological** Variability absent, decelerations present

A. Overview:
1. Most fetuses who later develop neurological handicap apparently do not show abnormal FHR patterns.
2. Compelling relationship between chronic patterns and CP.
3. Mechanical events may play a contributory role.
4. Doubtful relationship between ongoing or severe hypoxia and neurological injury.

B. Features of FHR patterns:
1. Rest-activity cycles—usually absent.
2. Baseline heart rate:
   a. Usually stable.
   b. Usually in high average range.
   c. Occasionally tachycardia or bradycardia—if heart involved.
3. Baseline variability:
   a. Usually absent.
   b. Sometimes exaggerated—"sawtooth pattern."
4. Accelerations:
   a. Usually absent.
   b. Isolated, bizarre in appearance.
   c. Do not coalesce.
5. Decelerations:
   a. Often absent.
   b. Variable decelerations with overshoot (chronic distress) is the most common deceleration.
   c. Bizarre/atypical decelerations.

C. EFM pattern of chronic distress:
1. Features—all must apply:
   a. Persistently absent variability.
   b. Variable decelerations with overshoot.
   c. Usually stable baseline rate.
2. Statistics (preliminary):
   a. About 0.25% of all tracings.
      (1) About a third are injured.
      (2) About a third die.
      (3) About a third are anomalous.
      (4) Rare intact survival.
   b. About 50% of all tracings of malpractice cases involve brain damage.
3. Clinically:
   a. Postdate or "dysmature" common.
   b. Thick meconium.
   c. Oligohydramnios.
   d. Maternal complaints of decreased fetal movement.
   e. Most have reactive NST in week before labor.

13

D. EFM pattern in anencephalic, hydrocephalic:
1. Baseline usually in upper range of normal.
2. Variability usually absent.
3. Rarely exaggerated variability with bizarre decelerations and accelerations.

POSTTERM PREGNANCY

A. Definitions:
1. Prolonged pregnancy, postdatism, postterm:
   a. Gestation greater than 294 days from LNMP.
   b. Obstetrical diagnosis.
2. Postmaturity, dysmaturity, postmature syndrome: "Dysmaturity" associated with postterm pregnancy, neonatal diagnosis.
B. Incidence:
1. Postterm pregnancy:
   a. 42 weeks: 10%.
   b. 43 weeks: 3%.
2. Dysmaturity syndrome:
   a. 38 weeks: 2% to 6%.
   b. 42 weeks: 20%.
C. Associated problems:
1. Anxiety.
2. Increased fetal size and weight/macrosomia.
3. Decrease in amniotic fluid volume.
4. Fetal wasting, dysmaturity.
5. Meconium passage/meconium aspiration.
6. Increased need for cesarean section:
   a. Dystocia: failed induction, macrosomia.
   b. Fetal distress:
      (1) Oligohydramnios leading to cord compression.
      (2) Hypoxia.
7. Death, birth trauma, neurological handicap.
8. Congenital anomaly.
D. Deterioration in postdate pregnancy:
1. Nutritional placental insufficiency:
   a. Diminished AFV and fetal body water.
   b. Diminished cord turgor.
   c. Cord compression—variable decelerations.
2. Respiratory placental insufficiency.
   a. Hypoxia, late decelerations.
E. Principles of care—Antepartum:
1. Avoid fetal dysmaturity, optimize timing of delivery.
2. Establish accurate dates early in gestation:
   a. Careful history—early prenatal examination.
   b. Liberal use of ultrasound.

c. Regular follow-up, examination at 20 weeks.
d. Loss of weight, poor fundal growth late in pregnancy.
3. Careful selection for elective induction:
   a. Pregnancy at 42 weeks with "good dates."
   b. Inducible cervix (Bishop's score ≥9).
   c. All pregnancies beyond 42 weeks.
4. Begin testing before 42 weeks (around 287 days).
5. Fetal surveillance:
   a. For nutritional function (dysmaturity): AFV.
   b. For respiratory function:
      (1) Fetal heart rate testing (NST, CST).
      (2) Fetal biophysical profile.
      (3) Estriol.
F. Intrapartum management:
1. Observe for fetal distress.
2. Monitor labor progress (Friedman curve).
3. Avoid difficult delivery, birth trauma (large baby).
4. Prompt attention to meconium at delivery of head.
G. Controversies:
1. "Unripe" cervix: Induction vs. expectant vs. ripen cervix.
2. Fetal surveillance—NST/CST/prostaglandins/biophysical profile/AFV.
3. Previous cesarean section:
   a. Trial of labor.
   b. Elective cesarean section.

OUTCOME RESULTS

A. Generalities:
1. Various tests predict normal outcome well, much less accurate in predicting poor outcome.
2. Each test shows a relatively high false-positive rate (40% to 80%), but low false negative rates (1%).
3. "It is easy to make a good baby look bad, but difficult to make a bad baby look good."
4. Despite popularity of tests, varying:
   a. Details of the interpretation.
   b. Testing schemes.
   c. Management strategies.
      (1) NST alone.
      (2) CST alone.
      (3) BPP alone.
      (4) NST/AFV.
5. All improve perinatal morbidity and mortality.
6. Which testing scheme is superior remains unresolved:
   a. No controlled studies in various clinical conditions.

TABLE 3.
Electronic Fetal Monitoring Pattern Interpretation and Intervention

Category	Baseline Rate	Baseline Stable	Variability	Accelerations	Decelerations	Interpretation	Action	Comments
Reassuring	110–150	Stable	Average	Coalesce	Absent, sporadic with prematures	No fetal indication for intervention, normal neurological control of FHR, asphyxia absent	Repeat as clinically indicated	Reassuring tracing, sleep-wake cycles, prematures may demonstrate small variable decelerations with movement
Suspicious Baseline	>150 <110	Stable	Decreased Average/ increased	Coalesce	Absent	Absent asphyxia—fetal provocation Postdate	Continue CTG, attempt to define cause; intervention may be necessary; anticipate normal outcome	Abnormal baseline, no decelerations; absent asphyxia; consider oligohydramnios, IUGR, fever, other remediable distress
Suspicious Variability	110–150 Any	Stable	Decreased Silent Sinusoidal	Absent	Absent Isolated, don't coalesce	Altered neurological control of FHR Asphyxia absent	Continue CTG, attempt to define cause; potential need to intervene; wide range of outcome	Abnormal neurological control; consider: prematurity, anomaly, neurological insult, drugs; if sinusoidal, consider fetal anemia
Threatening	110–150	Stable/ rising*	Average to increased	Usually present, coalesce	Late, variable,* prolonged*	Potential fetal asphyxia—early, normal neurological control of FHR	Correct problem, continue CTG, intervene if pattern deteriorates	Consider oligohydramnios, fetal breathing, early distress pushing (second stage)
Pathological	>150 / 110–150	Stable/ rising	Silent / Sinusoidal†	Absent	Late, variable† / Prolonged†	Fetal asphyxia—not compensated / Potential neurological handicap	Consider immediate intervention	Potentially reversible distress, e.g., diabetic ketoacidosis, excessive pushing (second stage)
Ominous Agonal	110–150 <110	Unstable,	Silent Sinusoidal falling†	Absent	Variable, late† Prolonged, atypical†	Fetal asphyxia—decompensated Potential neurological handicap, death imminent	Immediate intervention	Agonal tracing; imminent death

*Recovers to normal rate and variability.
†Does not recover to normal rate and variability.

b. Differences in methodology, test criteria, intervention strategy.
7. Normal test results do not guarantee normal outcome.

B. Benefits of NST/AFV scheme:
1. Availability—office procedure.
2. Minimal inconvenience, average time: 10 to 30 minutes.
3. Minimal need for additional or repeat testing.
4. Less subjective, fewer equivocal results.
5. Poses no risks or contraindications.
6. Provides additional information:
   a. Placental localization.
   b. Fetal presentation.
   c. Anomalies, etc.
7. BPP better than CST in discriminating NR NST.

C. False-normal test results:
1. Definition—death, poor outcome or late decelerations within one week of a normal test.
2. Incidence:
   a. NST—about 1% of reactive NST.
   b. CST—about 1% to 3% of negative CST.
   c. BPP—probably lower.
3. Etiology:
   a. Rapid deterioration of the fetus.
   b. Cord accident or abruptio placentae.
   c. Moribund fetus (CST only).
   d. Acute fetal or placental disorder.
   e. Trauma.
   f. Long interval after testing.
   g. Technical—spurious accelerations.
   h. Majority related to unpredictable factors.
4. Misinterpretation or failure to act on variable decelerations.

D. False-abnormal test results:
1. Definition—normal outcome after an abnormal test.
2. Incidence:
   a. NST—about 80% to 90%, i.e., most nonreactive NST fetuses have normal outcome.
   b. CST—about 50% of patients with positive CST who are allowed to labor.
   c. BPP—probably less than above.

3. Etiology:
   1. Technical.
   2. Supine position.
   3. Medication, especially phenobarbital, propanolol.
   4. "Excessive" stimulation.
   5. Alteration of fetal well-being.
   6. Other factors, e.g., smoking, fetal breathing (CST), variability (NST), tachycardia (NST).
   7. Test protocol—some babies have sleep-wake cycles longer than 20 to 40 minutes.
   8. Benefit of intervention.

CONCLUSIONS

A. Antepartum and intrapartum monitoring are associated with improved outcome and increased cesarean section rate.
B. Improvement in outcome is independent of antepartum test results or treatment or consistency of intrapartum interpretation.
C. Increased cesarean section rate is independent of antepartum test results or treatment but may be influenced by interpretation of EFM patterns.
D. Improved outcome statistics and increased section rate prevail as long as the patient is enrolled in an organized program of perinatal care.
E. Early intervention avoids fetal morbidity but increases risk of unnecessary intervention.
F. Irrespective of test, benefit to more frequent testing and liberalized criteria for intervention.
G. Including fetal evaluation in the assessment of risk improves outcome of both high- and low-risk pregnancies.
H. The evaluation of EFM tracings involves an analysis of the potential for asphyxia as well as fetal behavior.
I. Perinatal asphyxia does not mean that the fetus was injured.
J. Perinatal injury does not mean that the fetus was asphyxiated.
K. Injury from asphyxia, an uncommon event, does not mean that the injury was reasonably preventable.

TRACINGS

TRACING: 1

CLINICAL: Routine testing.

WEEKS: 41

RATE: 120

STV: Average.

LTV: Average.

DECELERATIONS: Absent.

ACCELERATIONS: Sporadic, coalesced.

UC: Occasional.

NST: Reactive.

CST: Negative.

OUTCOME: Normal.

COMMENT: In this reactive NST of the term fetus, the accelerations that begin at 6M are preceded by diminished variability and absent accelerations. The first set of accelerations arise out of decreased variability, but thereafter arise out of normal variability. This series of accelerations, the first one coupled, is followed by several more isolated accelerations, then a series of coalesced accelerations that mimic a transient tachycardia. The initial part of the coalesced acceleration at 18M contains a scalloped pattern that contains the suggestion of a return to baseline. This pattern occasionally may look like small variables with over-shoot but should be discounted as having any ominous importance in this context. Thereafter, the simulation of tachycardia is sustained for about 4 to 5 minutes before the heart rate returns to its previous baseline rate and variability. The duration of such coalesced accelerations varies from a few minutes to as long as 10–20 minutes and sometimes even longer. Immediately after this rapid flurry of accelerations and movements, the fetus, perhaps tired from the exertion, returns to the quiescent state to "sleep it off."

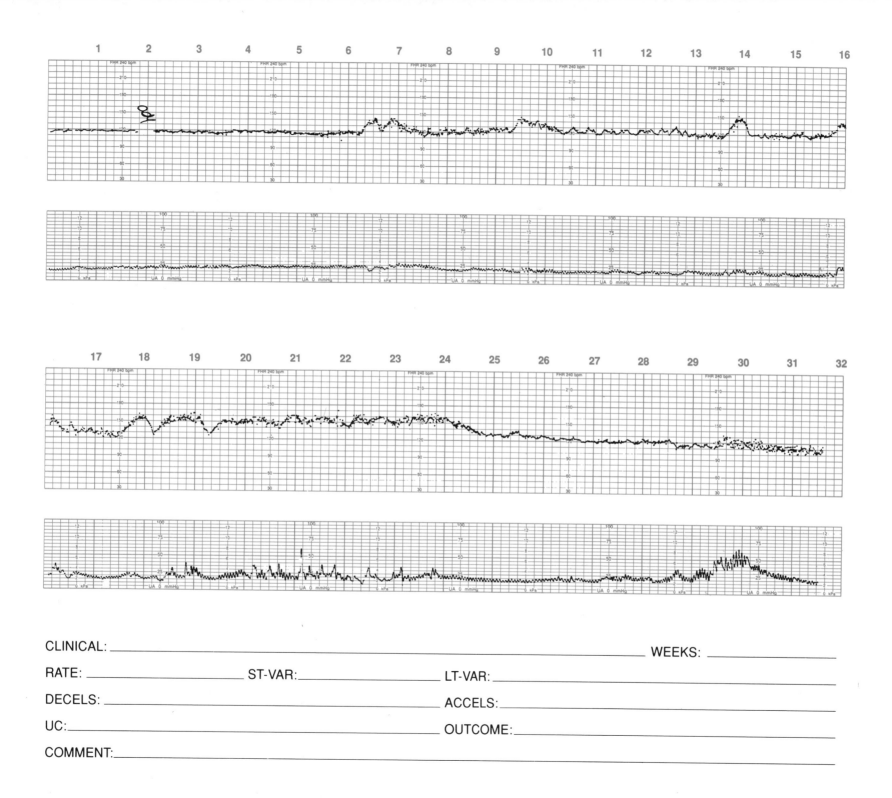

CLINICAL: _____   WEEKS: _____

RATE: _____ ST-VAR: _____ LT-VAR: _____

DECELS: _____ ACCELS: _____

UC: _____ OUTCOME: _____

COMMENT: _____

TRACING: 2

CLINICAL: Maternal hypertension.

WEEKS: 36

RATE: 120–130

STV: Average.

LTV: Average.

DECELERATIONS: Absent.

ACCELERATIONS: Frequent, sporadic.

UC: Low amplitude, occasional Braxton-Hicks.

NST: Reactive.

CST: Negative.

OUTCOME: Normal outcome.

COMMENT: This tracing illustrates a number of features of the reactive NST. During the first 16 minutes of the tracing the FHR exhibits no accelerations and minimal variability. If such a response were prolonged, the tracing would be classified as nonreactive and suggest abnormality. This epoch, which represents the sleep-rest phase of the sleep-wake cycle, offers few clues to the subsequent reactivity. Reactivity does not begin cataclysmically. Often the fetus has a few tentative accelerations that arise before the baseline variability increases. Thereafter, baseline variability increases and accelerations continue, initially isolated and then coalesced. Ultimately, the fetus re-enters the sleep cycle. Indeed, sleep-wake cycles may persist into early labor—spontaneous or induced.

The UC channel exhibits both high frequency, low amplitude oscillations along with low frequency, high amplitude uterine contractions (Braxton-Hicks). Although here more contractions appear during the reactive phase than the sleep cycle, this relationship is not consistent. Also, uterine contractions do not seem to modify the sleep-wake cycles of the fetus. This is a reassuring test in a mature baby with a baseline rate near the low end of the normal range.

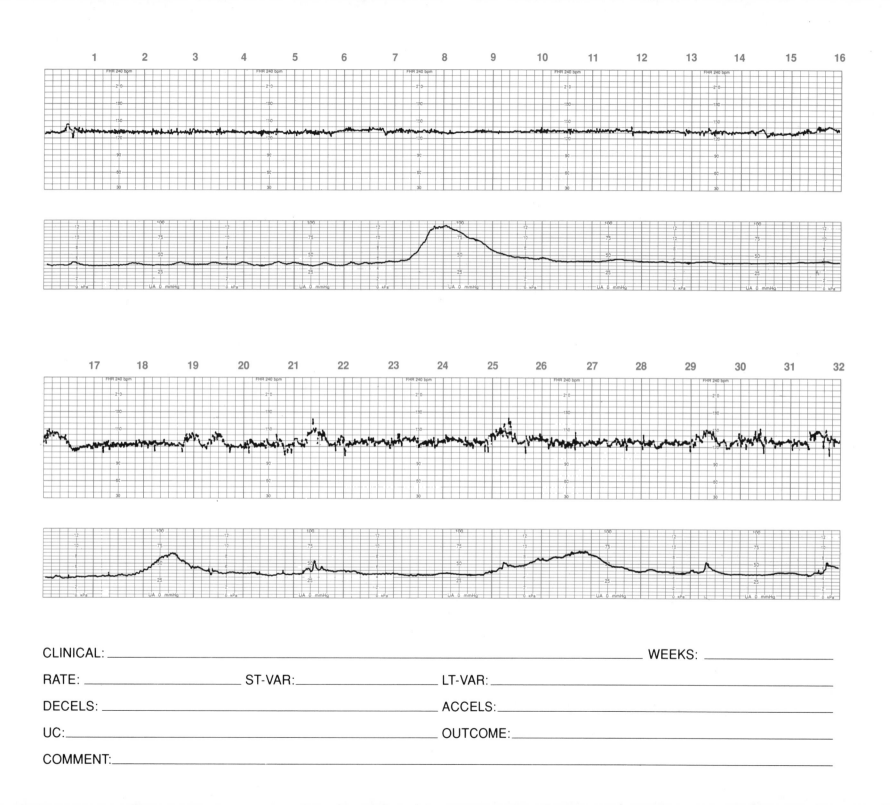

CLINICAL: _____ WEEKS: _____

RATE: _____ ST-VAR: _____ LT-VAR: _____

DECELS: _____ ACCELS: _____

UC: _____ OUTCOME: _____

COMMENT: _____

TRACING: 3

CLINICAL: Upper: Active fetus, maternal anxiety.
Lower: Atropine administration.

WEEKS: 41

BASELINE RATE: Upper: 140–150   Lower: 155–160

STV: Upper: Average. Lower: Absent.

LTV: Upper: Average. Lower: Decreased.

DECELERATIONS: Absent.

ACCELERATIONS: Upper: Abundant. Lower: Isolated.

UC: Upper: Occasional—mostly fetal movements.
Lower: 4½ to 7 minutes.

OUTCOME: Normal infant.

COMMENT: *Upper:* This tracing reveals a baseline rate of about 140–150 bpm and abundant accelerations which exceed 50 or 60 bpm. The accelerations tend to be somewhat irregular, lasting from less than a minute to more than minutes. They vary only slightly in terms of amplitude. The temptation to consider these changes as decelerations should be resisted. There is minimal uterine activity but abundant fetal movement which appears in flurries coincident with the accelerations above them. The baseline rate of 140–150 bpm cannot be determined until the tracing is 5–8 minutes old. Large accelerations are occasionally seen in fetal monitoring tracings. They usually are associated with relatively low baselines. Irrespective of the baseline rate, large accelerations bode no ominous importance.

Lower: This tracing, with a slightly higher baseline, reveals the effect of atropine (or scopolamine) on a normal fetus. Note that while the uterine activity, baseline, and periodic changes remain intact, the short-term variability is essentially eliminated. By inhibiting vagal activity, atropine decreases the variability, minimizes decelerations, and raises the heart rate. But atropine also uncovers periodic accelerations—the fetal sympathetic activity that accompanies uterine contractions.

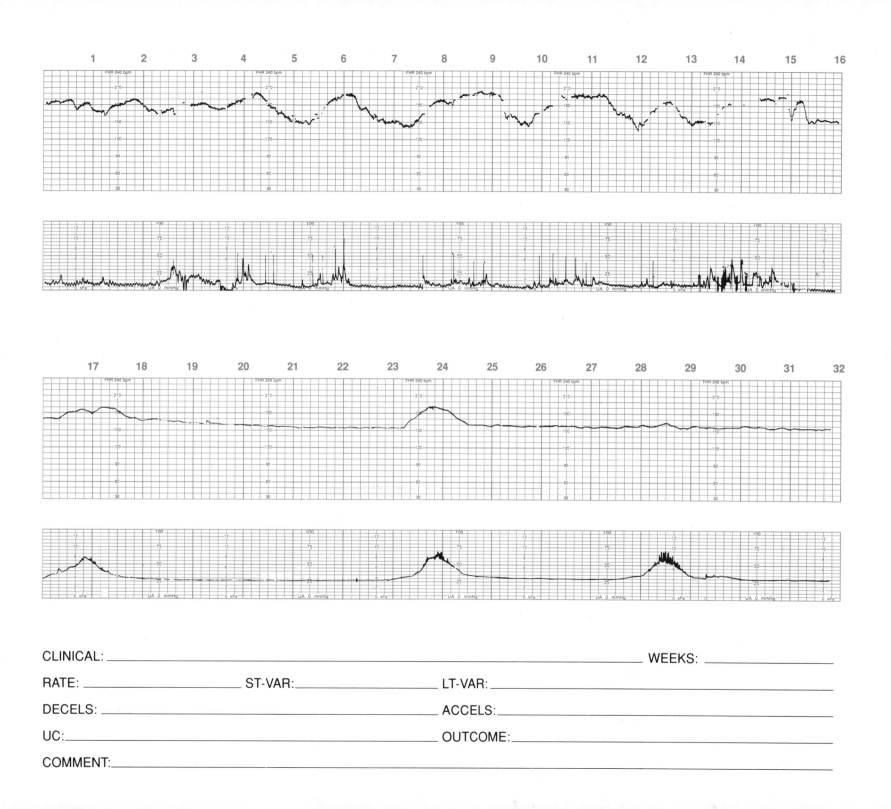

CLINICAL:_____ WEEKS:_____

RATE:_____ ST-VAR:_____ LT-VAR:_____

DECELS:_____ ACCELS:_____

UC:_____ OUTCOME:_____

COMMENT:_____

TRACING: 4

CLINICAL: Both: Routine testing.

WEEKS: 40

RATE: A: 120–130!   B: 130–140

STV: Both: Average.

LTV: Both: Average.

DECELERATIONS: Both: Absent.

ACCELERATIONS: Both: Abundant.

UC: A: Few, if any. B: Irregular.

NST: Both: Reactive.

CST: A: Insufficient data. B: Negative.

OUTCOME: Both: Normal.

COMMENT: *Upper panel* reveals a reactive NST but also contains the potential for misinterpreting the tracing as a series of decelerations. Indeed, the infant spends much more of its time accelerating than it does at the baseline. This panel contains no decelerations. Deciphering these changes requires an awareness of the abundant fetal movements and the absence of contractions. Note also that there is no obvious pattern or consistency to these "decelerations" which always return to the same baseline rate and variability despite marked variation in their duration.

In *lower panel,* variability and accelerations are associated with apparent fetal movement. Several of the accelerations, at 25M and 30M, return to the baseline with a slight undershooting of the baseline, the so-called *lambda* pattern. This pattern is of no consequence and should not be confused with a deceleration.

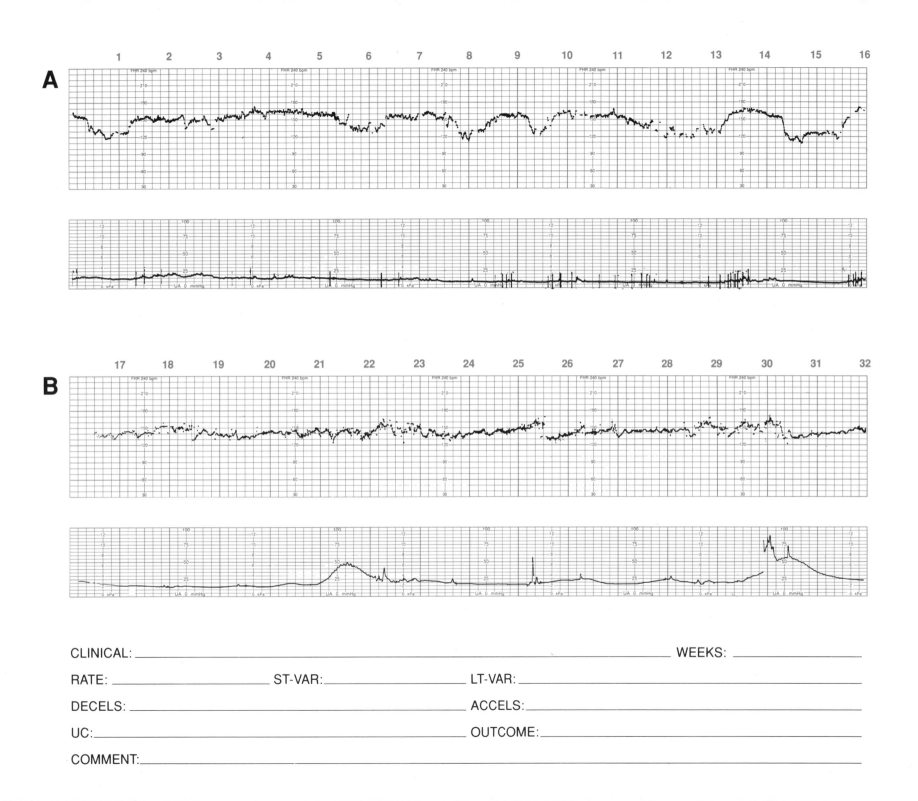

CLINICAL: _____   WEEKS: _____

RATE: _____ ST-VAR: _____   LT-VAR: _____

DECELS: _____   ACCELS: _____

UC: _____   OUTCOME: _____

COMMENT: _____

TRACING: 5

CLINICAL: Upper: NST. Lower: Labor.

WEEKS: 41

BASELINE RATE: Upper: 120   Lower: 160

STV: Upper: Average. Lower: Decreased.

LTV: Upper: Exaggerated. Lower: Decreased.

DECELERATIONS: None.

ACCELERATIONS: Upper: Coalesced. Lower: None.

UC: Irregular.

OUTCOME: Normal.

COMMENT: The *upper panel* reflects normal to increased baseline variability and numerous epochal fetal movements during an NST in the prodromal phase of labor. Note that the movements appear in groups and that many of the accelerations coalesce. Note the frequent fetal movements at the bottom of the FHR grid. The almost rampant changes in the heart rate should not be interpreted as decelerations (10M and 14M). These represent a return to the fetal baseline (3M). This is quite a reassuring NST.

The *lower panel* was obtained from the same fetus later in labor after the administration of narcotic to the mother. The diminished variability is punctuated by rather discrete accelerations and nondescript, minimal decelerations which bear no consistent relationship to the irregular uterine contractions. This change in the fetal pattern represents *drug effect*, not asphyxia.

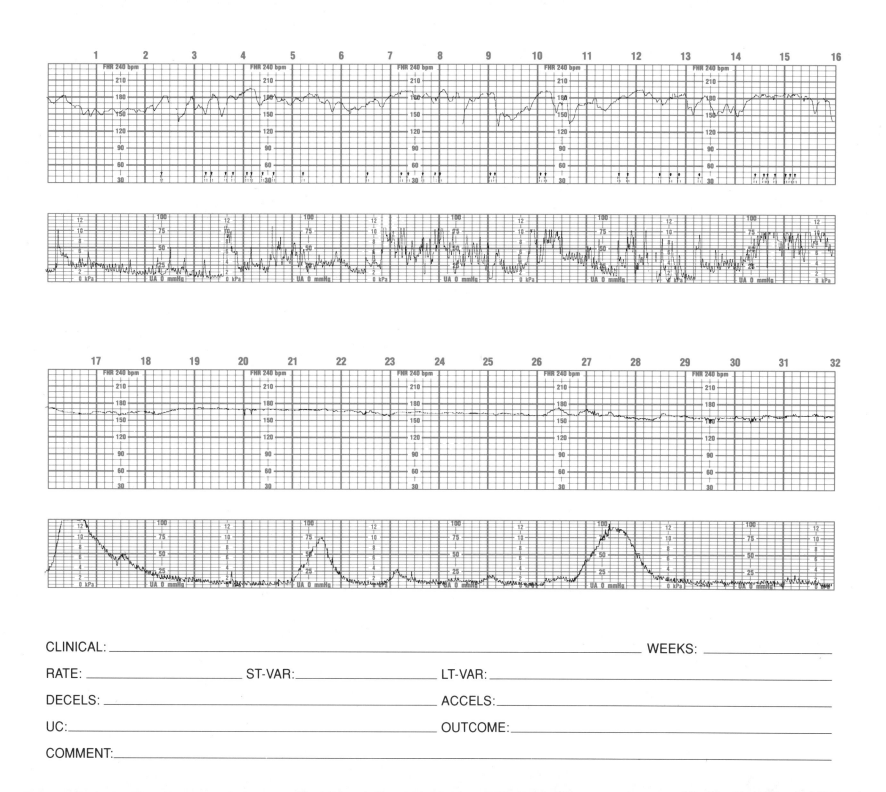

CLINICAL: _____ WEEKS: _____

RATE: _____ ST-VAR: _____ LT-VAR: _____

DECELS: _____ ACCELS: _____

UC: _____ OUTCOME: _____

COMMENT: _____

TRACING: 6

CLINICAL: Routine testing.

WEEKS: 38

RATE: Upper: 160–170   Lower: 190

STV: Decreased.

LTV: Decreased.

DECELERATIONS: Mild variable.

ACCELERATIONS: Multiple sporadic.

UC: Occasional.

NST: Reactive.

CST: Negative.

OUTCOME: Normal.

COMMENT: This unusual tracing contains considerable potential for misinterpretation. At the outset, establishing a baseline is somewhat difficult. The reader has to decide whether these obvious changes in the heart rate represent accelerations or decelerations. To represent decelerations the baseline heart rate would in fact have to be well over 200 bpm. While the amplitude of such "decelerations" would range from 30 to 50 bpm, the duration and shape are inconsistent among themselves, and inconsistent with any known pattern of decelerations. More reasonably, these represent a series of accelerations with a baseline rate of 160 to 170 bpm. The evidence for this includes the irregularity of the pattern and the consistent relationship to movement on the UC channel. The pattern is unusual in that large accelerations generally arise from lower baseline heart rates. That is, the higher the baseline the smaller the amplitude of accelerations. High amplitude accelerations, greater than 50 bpm, have no known significance. The lower panel from the same baby is more characteristic of a reactive fetus with baseline tachycardia. Here the rate is so high and variability so diminished that the usual features accompanying accelerations are not seen. Such patterns may be seen in febrile patients or occasionally in cocaine-addicted mothers. This tracing bears some resemblance to the pattern of fetal injury.

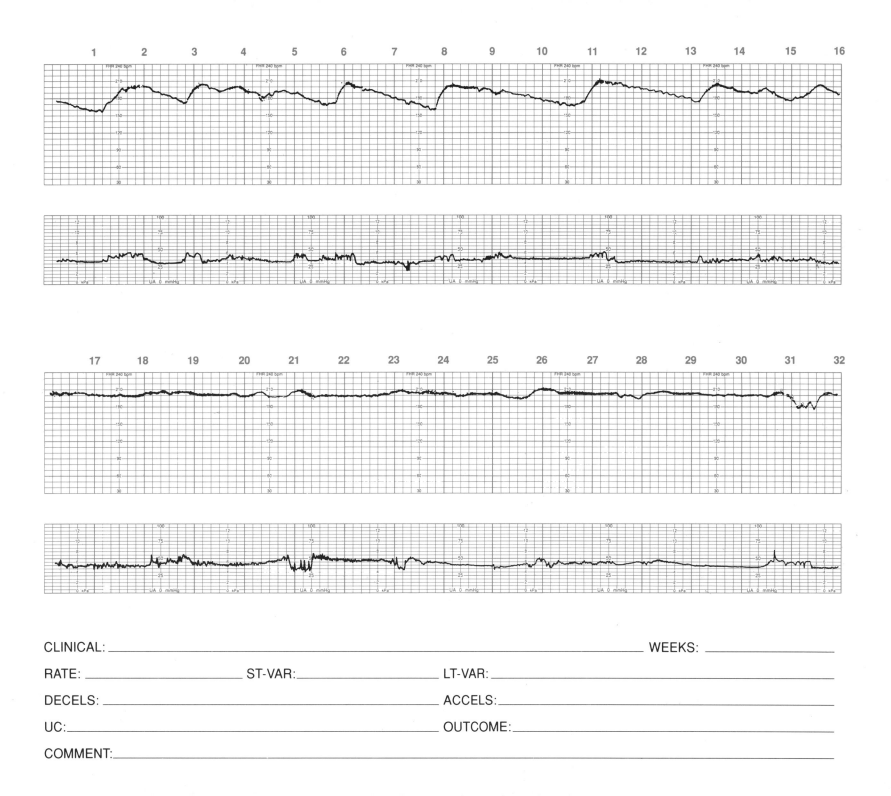

CLINICAL: _____ WEEKS: _____

RATE: _____ ST-VAR: _____ LT-VAR: _____

DECELS: _____ ACCELS: _____

UC: _____ OUTCOME: _____

COMMENT: _____

TRACING: 7

CLINICAL: Both: Early labor.

WEEKS: 40

RATE: A: 120   B: 140

STV: Both: Average.

LTV: Both: Average? Sinusoidal.

DECELERATIONS: Both: Absent.

ACCELERATIONS: A: Abundant sporadic. B: Absent.

UC: Both: Early labor, irregular.

NST: A: Reactive. B: Nonreactive.

CST: Both: Negative.

OUTCOME: Both: Normal.

COMMENT: Both of these tracings are or were preceded by unequivocal reactivity. In the upper panel we see the evolution from a reactive NST with frequent, even sustained accelerations, into a regular oscillating pattern (not sinusoidal) characteristic of fetal sucking. These oscillations are somewhat irregular, more rounded at the top, more irregular and less rounded at the bottom. There is obvious diminution in fetal activity during the second half of this panel compared to the first half. Normally, when the fetus breathes it does not move, and vice versa. The appearance of either a "sinusoidal" or oscillating pattern in association with reactivity elsewhere is of no consequence whatsoever and almost certainly bespeaks fetal activity despite frequent contractions.

The *lower panel* was obtained during early labor following the administration of the narcotic, alphaprodine. Under the influence of the medication, this pattern evolves into a regular sinusoidal pattern. Here the frequency of the oscillations is greater than those above, though the amplitude is less. Also there is greater irregularity at the bottom of the oscillations than at the top. The pattern prevails despite the mild decelerations at 24M and 29M that describe no consistent pattern. The sinusoidal pattern appears about 10 to 30 minutes after administration and may last up to 2 hours. The undulations tend to be somewhat irregular, and may be affected readily by uterine contractions and reversed by naloxone (Narcan). They are not ominous.

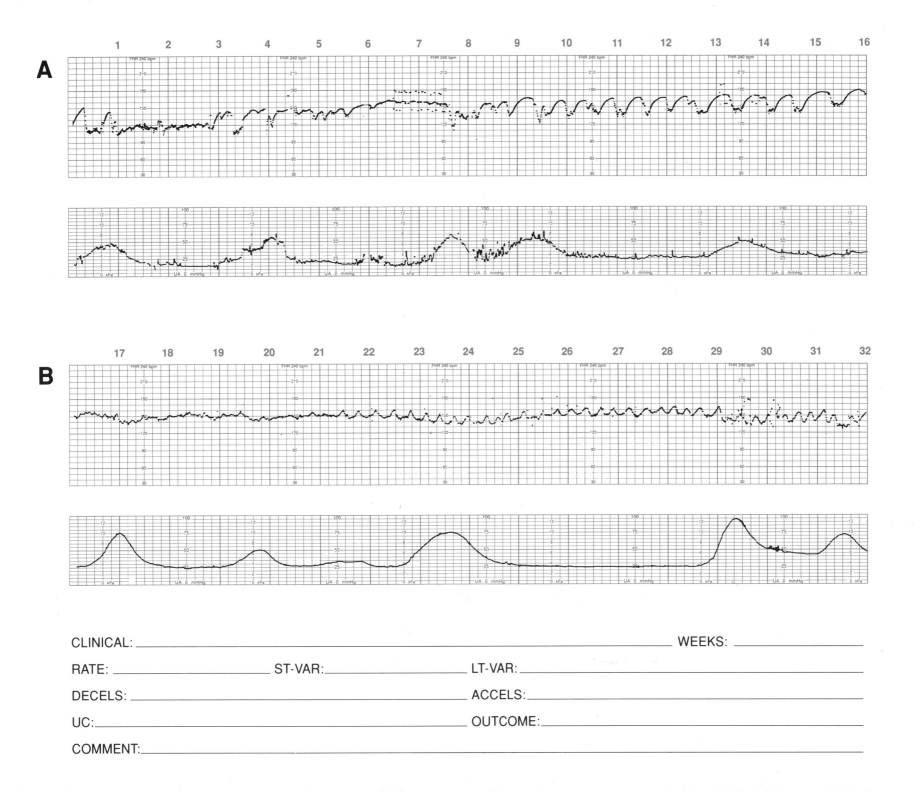

CLINICAL: _____ WEEKS: _____

RATE: _____ ST-VAR: _____ LT-VAR: _____

DECELS: _____ ACCELS: _____

UC: _____ OUTCOME: _____

COMMENT: _____

TRACING: 8

CLINICAL: Poor maternal weight gain.

WEEKS: A: 38   B: 39

RATE: 130–140

STV: Both: Average.

LTV: Both: Average, at least.

DECELERATIONS: Both: Absent.

ACCELERATIONS: Both: Abundant, but short-lived.

UC: Both: Occasional.

NST: Functionally reactive–too reactive.

CST: Negative.

OUTCOME: Normal infant (short-term evaluation).

COMMENT: These tracings were obtained from the same fetus about 1 week apart. Both tests are clearly reactive with abundant accelerations, obvious variability, and no decelerations. These tracings are unusual, however, in that there are no sleep cycles—this "wired fetus" is always awake. Such tracings may be seen in mothers with cocaine addiction (as in this case) or other addictions. Such addiction does not compromise the oxygen availability of the baby but may in fact create disturbances in fetal growth as well as fetal sleep-wake patterns (behavior). Similar tracings, which show reactivity but without obvious sleep cycles, may also be seen in nonaddicted mothers who have undergone some stress, such as automobile accidents in which there is no harm to the fetus.

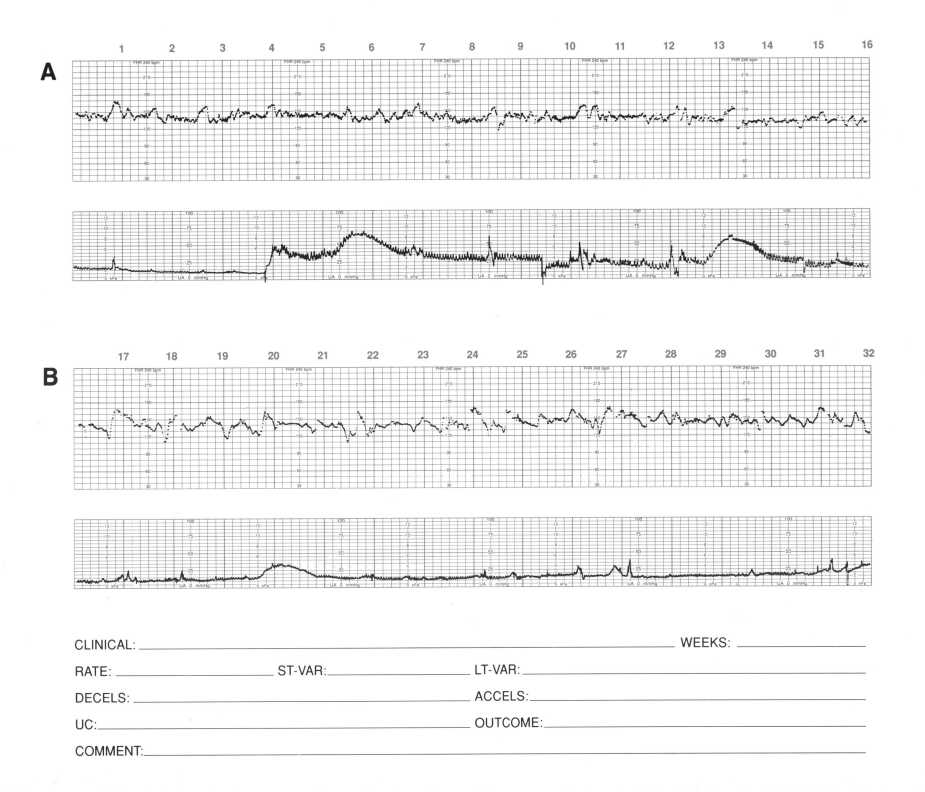

CLINICAL: _____ WEEKS: _____

RATE: _____ ST-VAR:_____ LT-VAR: _____

DECELS: _____ ACCELS:_____

UC:_____ OUTCOME:_____

COMMENT:_____

TRACING: 9

CLINICAL: Term. Possible IUGR.

WEEKS: 37

RATE: 140–160

STV: Decreased.

LTV: Decreased.

DECELERATIONS: None.

ACCELERATIONS: Overshoot.

UC: Early labor.

OUTCOME: Normal, IUGR.

COMMENT: This previously normal tracing reveals a rapid rise in heart rate (>50 bpm) over about 8 minutes, unaccompanied by decelerations. Few factors can change the rate this dramatically and asphyxia is not one of them. This rapid a rise is also unlikely to be the result of maternal fever (excluding chills) or beta-mimetic drugs, which elevate the rate much more leisurely. Profound asphyxia would induce bradycardia, not tachycardia. Lesser degrees of asphyxia during labor would produce more obvious late decelerations and eventually a modest elevation in rate—rarely as dramatic as this. Atropine and cholinergic blockade could change the rate this rapidly but they rarely induce tachycardia above 155 to 170 bpm. Arrhythmia in the form of paroxysmal tachycardia tends to develop far more rapidly, usually over several heart beats.

In this case, the mother had been given a narcotic (meperidine) and became dysphoric, anxious, and then vomited. The fetal heart rate changes seen here developed immediately thereafter. How best to explain this tracing? For want of better explanation, this is "fetal anxiety." Note that the entire episode lasts about 30 minutes. Although an effect of nalorphine (Naline) administered at 15M cannot be excluded, this sequence of events has been seen without the addition of the narcotic antagonist.

During the tachycardia the variability is markedly diminished with small accelerations and decelerations suggesting overshoot related to the diminution in parasympathetic tone. The pattern subsides in 20 to 30 minutes. If narcotics have not induced the pattern, they are frequently effective in bringing the rate down. This is *not* an asphyxial episode. Note the exaggerated maternal breathing pattern during contractions after the narcotic has been neutralized.

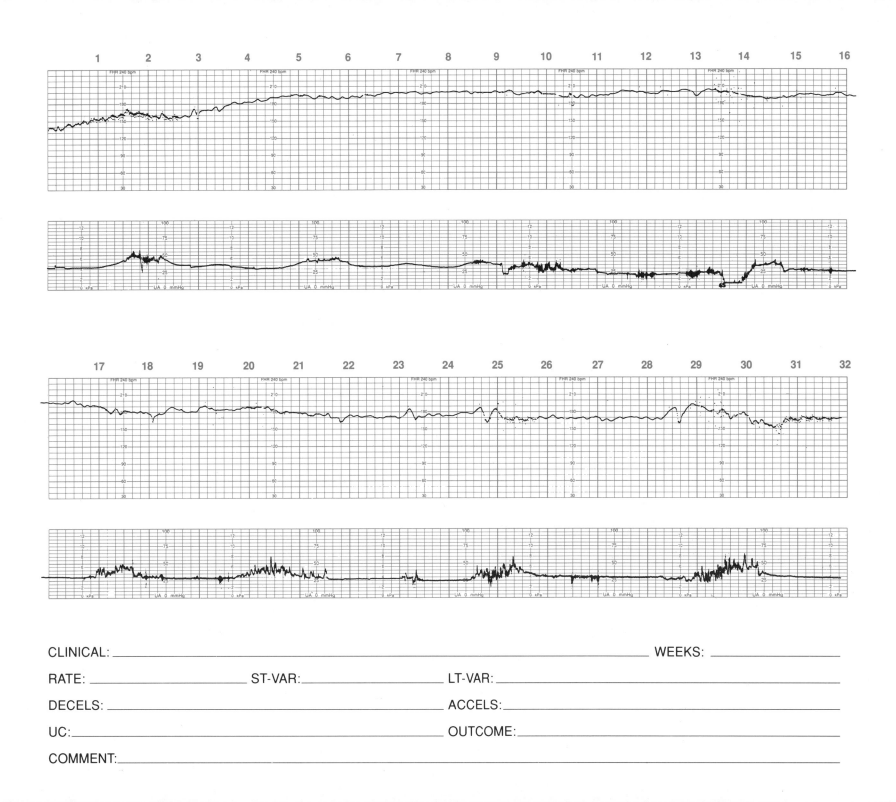

CLINICAL: _____ WEEKS: _____

RATE: _____ ST-VAR: _____ LT-VAR: _____

DECELS: _____ ACCELS: _____

UC: _____ OUTCOME: _____

COMMENT: _____

TRACING: 10

CLINICAL: Both: Decreased fetal movements.

WEEKS: Both: 41

RATE: Both: 140–150

STV: Both: Decreased.

LTV: Both: Decreased.

DECELERATIONS: Both: Absent.

ACCELERATIONS: Both: Sporadic.

UC: A: Absent. B: With provocation.

OUTCOME: Both: Normal.

COMMENT: These tracings illustrate features of the intermediate NST. Although the *upper panel* contains abundant accelerations, these accelerations, apparently associated with FM, do not fulfill the criteria for reactivity. These accelerations are associated with decreased baseline variability, and tend to be isolated and of minimal amplitude. Although there is no evidence that the fetus is now compromised, this tracing should not be dismissed as reactive. In this case the infant's prematurity is the likely explanation of the pattern.

The *lower panel* represents an attempt to stimulate the fetus using abdominal palpation. Note at 22M the immediate response of the fetal heart to the provocation but the absence of any sustained response. It is a proper response for a responsive fetus but should not be regarded as a reactive NST. Most provocation maneuvers, including palpation and the administration of glucose,

may shorten, to a small degree, the amount of time needed to perform the NST. Practically, these gentle provocations do not change the sleep-wake cycles, although, as in this case, they may provoke an acceleration. Only the acoustic stimulation shows obvious potential for changing the normal sleep-wake pattern of the infant. It may do this by the inducement of pain—a dubious approach.

The intermediate NST pattern may result from prematurity, temporary excitement or stress in the mother, maternal medication, or deterioration of the fetal condition. Given this test result, the well-being of the fetus should be further evaluated with the biophysical profile or by extending the NST. When the fetus is premature, it may reasonably be interpreted as a normal response unless obvious reactive patterns have been seen earlier in this fetus.

An intrapartum fetal death within 20 minutes of a reassuring acoustically stimulated fetal heart rate acceleration has been reported. The cause of death in this instance was congenital pneumonia, gram-negative sepsis, and meconium aspiration. Umbilical cord pH values obtained at delivery did not demonstrate asphyxia (i.e., low pO_2, high pCO_2, and low pH), but suggested a metabolic acidosis typical of sepsis.

REFERENCES

Strong TH Jr, Masaki DI, Sarno AP, et al: Fetal death from sepsis following a reassuring intrapartum fetal acoustic stimulation test. *Obstet Gynecol* 1989; 74(suppl 2):465–468.
Strong TH Jr, Masaki DI, Sarno AP, et al: Fetal death from sepsis following a reassuring intrapartum fetal acoustic stimulation test [reply]. *Obstet Gynecol* 1990; 75:307–308.

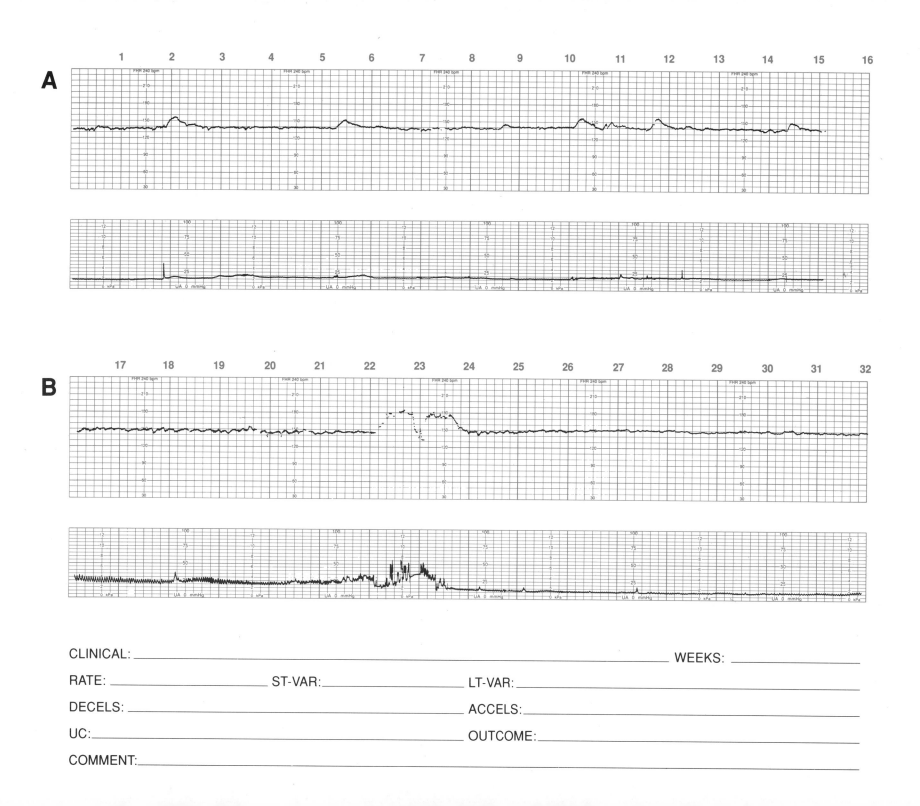

CLINICAL: _____ WEEKS: _____

RATE: _____ ST-VAR: _____ LT-VAR: _____

DECELS: _____ ACCELS: _____

UC: _____ OUTCOME: _____

COMMENT: _____

TRACING: 11

CLINICAL: Early labor.

WEEKS: Both: 40

RATE: Both: 160

STV: Both: Decreased.

LTV: Both: Decreased.

DECELERATIONS: Both: Absent.

ACCELERATIONS: Both: Sporadic.

UC: A: Irregular. B: Frequent.

NST: Both: Intermediate.

CST: Both: Negative.

OUTCOME: Both: Normal.

COMMENT: These two patterns focus on deviations from normal reactivity in the otherwise well fetus. In both tracings, the accelerations are not accompanied by normal variability. In the *upper panel,* the patient is receiving phenobarbital. The contractions produce minimal accelerations but no sustained variability or coalescence. Abdominal palpation at 9M produces an unequivocal acceleration, larger than that produced by the contraction, but no sustained reactivity.

The *lower panel* was obtained in labor following the administration of a narcotic, then epidural anesthesia. The head is high in the pelvis. Contractions induce brief, reasonably smooth accelerations but are unassociated with normal variability. Although this fetus is not asphyxiated, its reactivity is depressed, probably the result of the medications.

Normally, accelerations arise out of normal variability. They tend to recur in flurries, even without provocation, and often coalesce. If the fetus deteriorates, or has tachycardia, or is given barbiturates, the accelerations may remain but the additional features tend to disappear. Thus, accelerations may be isolated and unassociated with normal variability. They may still appear with provocation such as with contractions in the *lower panel.* These features do not speak for an asphyxiated baby or for one who is necessarily resilient and reactive. This sequence defines the intermediate pattern of the NST. It does not often represent fetal distress; "fetal malaise" seems a far more appropriate term. In this respect, caution must be exercised in interpreting the results of provocation with sound or stimulation. The results of these provocations may be judged reactive if they induce the entire pattern of reactivity, which includes variability and coalesced accelerations. The induction of single or isolated accelerations does not qualify as reactivity.

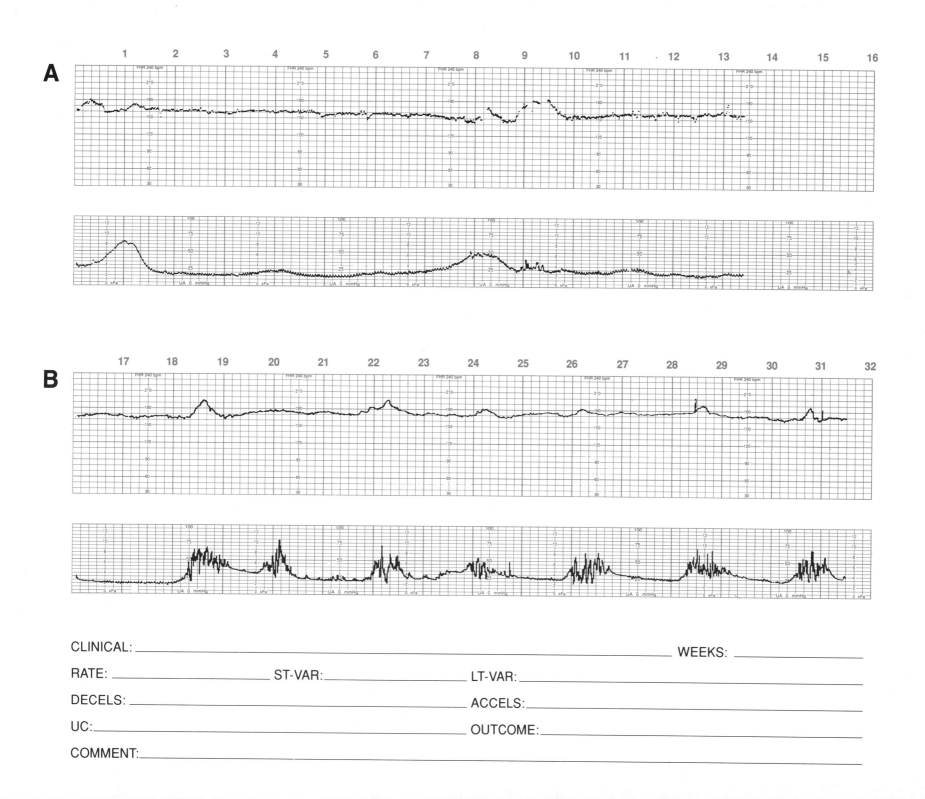

CLINICAL: _____ WEEKS: _____

RATE: _____ ST-VAR: _____ LT-VAR: _____

DECELS: _____ ACCELS: _____

UC: _____ OUTCOME: _____

COMMENT: _____

TRACING: 12

CLINICAL: Preterm labor.

WEEKS: 30

RATE: 150

STV: Decreased.

LTV: Average.

DECELERATIONS: Mild variable.

ACCELERATIONS: ?Overshoot.

UC: Irregular.

NST: Nonreactive.

CST: Negative.

OUTCOME: Premature birth; RDS.

COMMENT: This tracing was obtained from a pregnancy at 30 weeks' gestation immediately following an automobile accident. The tracing contains oscillations in the baseline rate (long-term variability), but minimal short-term variability. Note the stable baseline rate and obvious absence of reactivity. Decelerations are minimal and subscribe to no specific pattern. They show no relationship to the frequent uterine contractions. In this case, the mother was under considerable emotional distress from a recent automobile accident and had significant abdominal contusions. The pattern prompted concern for the condition of the baby as well as the potential for placental abruption. With continuous observation the uterine activity diminished and the heart rate pattern evolved into one with normal reactivity.

The analysis of this tracing is complicated by the gestational age as well as the anxiety and trauma visited on the patient. The frequent contractions raise the potential for placental abruption, but they are quite irregular in amplitude, duration, and interval. Contraction patterns associated with placental abruption tend to be far more consistent (see Tracing 17,A). The absence of significant decelerations in relationship to the contractions precludes significant hypoxia. This irregular pattern of a small acceleration and decelerations is typical of the active, premature fetus. It does bear a superficial resemblance to the chronic heart rate pattern seen on Tracing 59.

In addition to the above, maternal anxiety, with secretion of norepinephrine (a stimulant of uterine activity) may modify fetal heart rate and activity patterns. Fetuses may remain nonreactive, show occasional accelerations and minimal movements, or show variability, but few accelerations. If the fetus is injured, then reactivity will be significantly diminished and the baseline rate will likely be elevated. With injury decelerations are also common.

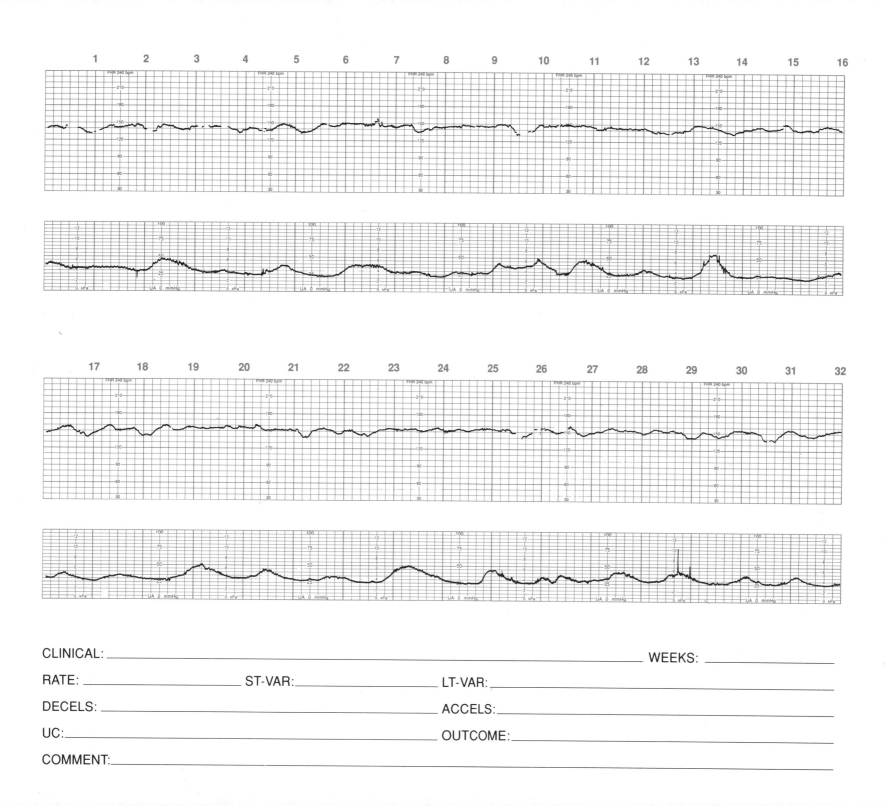

CLINICAL: _____ WEEKS: _____

RATE: _____ ST-VAR: _____ LT-VAR: _____

DECELS: _____ ACCELS: _____

UC: _____ OUTCOME: _____

COMMENT: _____

TRACING: 13

CLINICAL: Diabetes, class B.

WEEKS: 36

RATE: Upper: 150   Lower: 160

STV: Decreased.

LTV: Decreased to average.

DECELERATIONS: Absent.

ACCELERATIONS: Sporadic, frequent.

UC: Irregular.

NST: Reactive.

CST: Negative.

OUTCOME: Normal.

COMMENT: This tracing reveals a baseline tachycardia and, at least initially, occasional isolated accelerations that appear to be associated with fetal movement. Variability is diminished and the accelerations do not coalesce. The apparent, slight deceleration at 13M should be discounted. It likely represents fetal breathing movements (at the end of the contraction) or possibly a slightly delayed lambda pattern. The *lower panel* reveals the evolution of the reactive pattern with frequent accelerations and fetal movement. Amid the fetal activity between 26M and 27M we find small, variable decelerations. These are of no consequence and do not imply compromise or oligohydramnios. The half-deceleration seen at 23M+ is artifact. Because of technical limitations, external devices may erroneously create half-decelerations or half-accelerations sometimes associated with fetal movement as seen here. To qualify as an acceleration or deceleration, substantial segments of both the descending and ascending limbs must be seen.

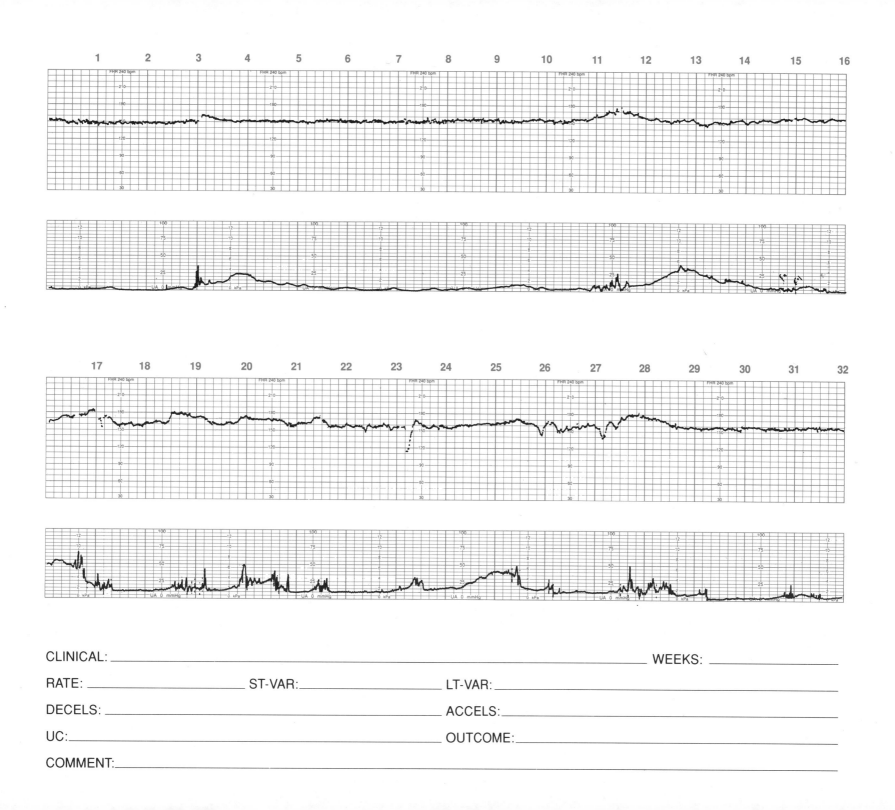

CLINICAL:_____ WEEKS:_____

RATE:_____ ST-VAR:_____ LT-VAR:_____

DECELS:_____ ACCELS:_____

UC:_____ OUTCOME:_____

COMMENT:_____

TRACING: 14

CLINICAL: Decreased fetal movement.

WEEKS: 30

RATE: 160

STV: Decreased.

LTV: Decreased.

DECELERATIONS: Absent.

ACCELERATIONS: Sporadic.

UC: Occasional, irregular.

NST: Nonreactive.

CST: Insufficient data.

OUTCOME: Preterm delivery; normal.

COMMENT: This tracing from a preterm fetus illustrates tachycardia, apparently decreased variability, with several brief, nonrepetitive, hard-to-classify decelerations. There are several accelerations of minimal amplitude at 8M, perhaps at 13M, and at 27M. The three contractions beginning at 26M elicit no obvious deceleration. The apparent decelerations at 8M and 28M represent the lambda pattern. Alternatively, the deceleration at 8M may simply represent a response to fetal movement in the preterm infant. The deceleration at 28M should not be overread as a "late deceleration." By definition, late decelerations are not initiated by accelerations. Similarly, late decelerations recur with subsequent contractions; this one does not. Although there is no obvious reactivity in this tracing, there are somewhat more oscillations ("variability") in the first 14 minutes than in the next 13 minutes. If the tracing were extended these epochal changes would continue to recur.

Over the subsequent weeks of testing, the heart rate decreased somewhat, the patterns of activity became more organized and associated with more obvious accelerations and rest-activity cycles. This pattern, therefore, abnormal by term standards, is quite common in pregnancies before 32 weeks and will eventually evolve into a mature, reactive pattern.

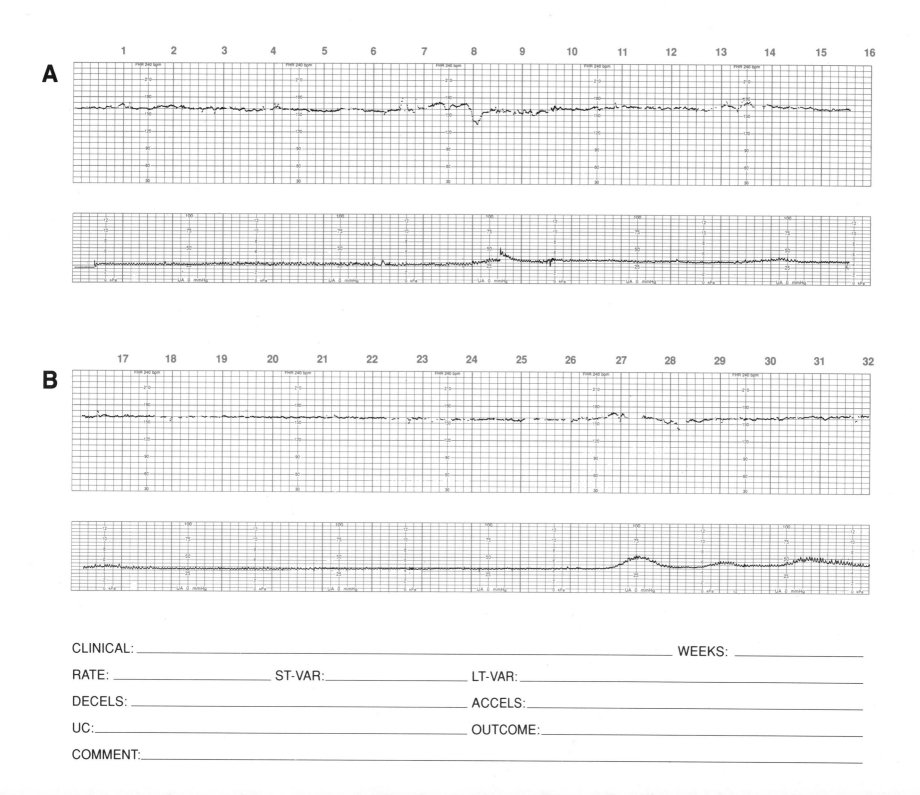

CLINICAL:_____ WEEKS:_____

RATE:_____ ST-VAR:_____ LT-VAR:_____

DECELS:_____ ACCELS:_____

UC:_____ OUTCOME:_____

COMMENT:_____

TRACING: 15

CLINICAL: Both: Decreased fetal movement.

WEEKS: Both: 33

RATE: A: 130   B: 160–170

STV: Both: Decreased.

LTV: Both: Absent.

DECELERATIONS: Both: Absent.

ACCELERATIONS: Both: Absent.

UC: A: Mild, irregular. B: High frequency, low amplitude.

NST: Both: Nonreactive.

CST: A: Negative. B: Unsatisfactory.

OUTCOME: Both: Subsequent normal tests and outcome.

COMMENT: Labeling a tracing as nonreactive warrants additional commentary lest follow-up testing be inappropriately delayed. These nonreactive tracings contain no obvious decelerations. Conventionally, such test results are deemed to require further testing in the form of the CST or profile. To some, such additional testing must be undertaken immediately. To others, further testing may wait until after a meal or overnight. What else can be said about these tracings beyond the obvious absence of accelerations, variability, or decelerations? Specifically, these nonreactive tracings fail to show such pathologic commentary as instability of the baseline, sinusoidal patterns, or small variable decelerations with overshoot. The absence of these features suggests that neither acute asphyxia nor imminent fetal death is likely.

The differential diagnosis includes: congenital anomaly, prolonged sleep state, premature fetus, maternal medication (e.g., phenobarbital). Several alternatives are available to refine the likely diagnosis. Either the NST may be prolonged, oxytocin may be infused, or a biophysical profile may be performed. In any case, allowing the patient some lunch is likely of little consequence. On the other hand, if the baseline rate were unstable or sinusoidal, or decelerations appeared, either spontaneously or associated with spontaneous contractions, then prompt further evaluation or delivery is required.

In the *upper panel* the UC channel reveals occasional contractions of minimal amplitude. The *lower panel* reveals high frequency, low amplitude uterine activity.

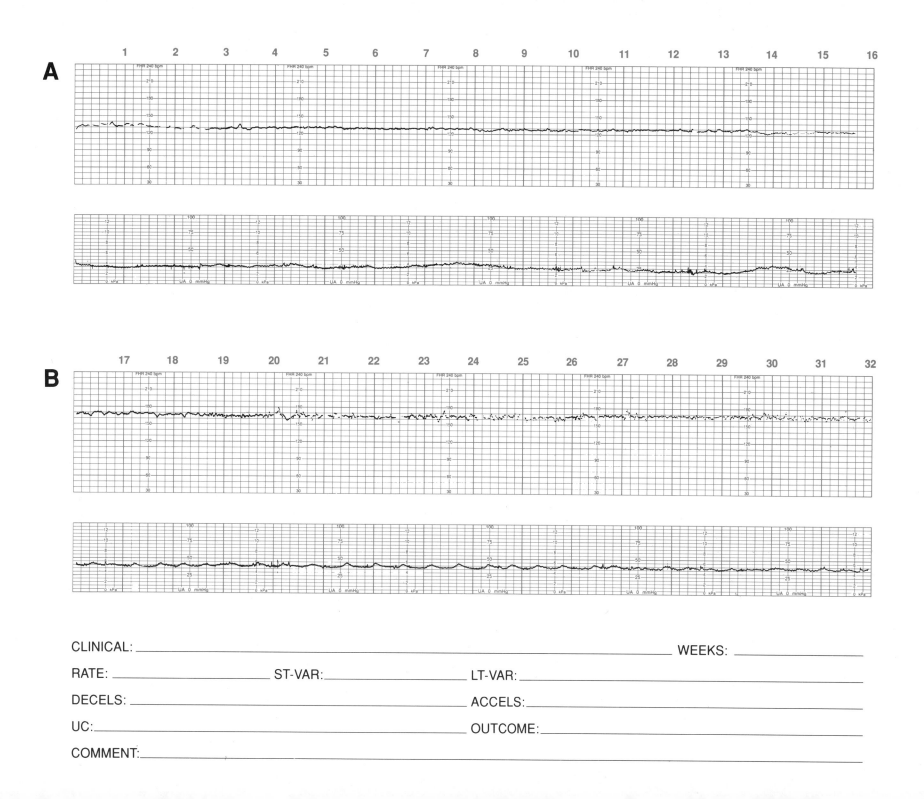

CLINICAL: _____ WEEKS: _____

RATE: _____ ST-VAR: _____ LT-VAR: _____

DECELS: _____ ACCELS: _____

UC: _____ OUTCOME: _____

COMMENT: _____

TRACING: 16

CLINICAL: A: Postdate. B: Decreased fetal movement.

WEEKS: A: 42. B: 38

RATE: Both: About 100.

STV: A: Average. B: Decreased.

LTV: A: Average. B: Decreased.

DECELERATIONS: Both: Absent!

ACCELERATIONS: A: Abundant, sporadic. B: Absent.

UC: A: Spontaneous. B: High frequency and Braxton-Hicks.

NST: A: Reactive. B: Nonreactive.

CST: Both: Negative.

OUTCOME: A: Normal. B: Congenital anomaly.

COMMENT: These two panels illustrate baseline bradycardia. In the *upper panel* we find obvious accelerations with considerable fetal movement and no decelerations with contractions. The apparent deceleration beyond 5M represents the lambda pattern rather than any significant deceleration. There is no hint of decelerations thereafter. The contractions are accompanied by abundant FM, usually at the beginning of the UC, associated with accelerations. The tracing also shows variability and should be considered reactive.

Modest degrees of baseline bradycardia with reactivity should provoke little concern. They are frequently associated with term or postterm pregnancies and do not represent hypoxia or compromise.

The *lower panel* reveals absent reactivity but no decelerations with the uterine contraction at 23M. The differential diagnosis of this heart rate pattern is broad. It may represent simply a prolonged sleep cycle, congenital heart block, or very remotely, hypothermia. As a generalization, fetuses with complete heart block show baseline rates between 60 and 80 bpm which are invariably nonreactive. They may have some modest oscillations around this baseline rate but obvious accelerations are rare. Another differential diagnosis is the presence of congenital or acquired neurologic abnormality. Anomalies account for a disproportionate share of abnormal antepartum tests. About 10%–20% of abnormal antepartum tests derive from fetuses with congenital anomaly. Anomalies, however, produce no consistent FHR patterns.

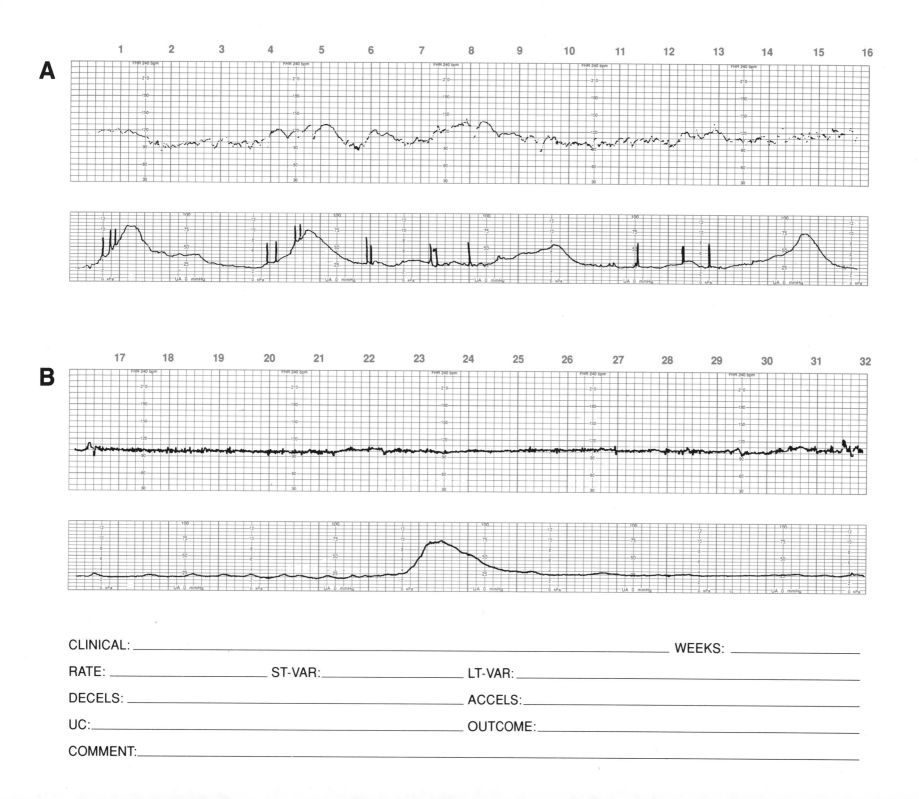

CLINICAL: _____ WEEKS: _____

RATE: _____ ST-VAR: _____ LT-VAR: _____

DECELS: _____ ACCELS: _____

UC: _____ OUTCOME: _____

COMMENT: _____

TRACING: 17

CLINICAL: A: Abdominal pain. B: Fever.

WEEKS: 36

RATE: A: 150   B: 155

STV: Both: Absent.

LTV: Both: Absent.

DECELERATIONS: Both: ?Late.

ACCELERATIONS: Both: Absent.

UC: A: Frequent, hypertonus. B: Frequent, irregular.

NST: A: Nonreactive. B: Nonreactive.

CST: Both: Suspicious.

OUTCOME: A: Normal. B: Neonatal sepsis.

COMMENT: These two examples of nonreactive NST invite the reader to decide whether late decelerations are also present. The easiest way to proceed is to cover the UC channel, then draw a line at the level of the baseline heart rate (about 160 bpm), parallel to the baseline. The line need only be above and close to the baseline. One then determines the presence or absence of a pattern of decelerations below the line which is regular in timing and consistent in configuration. Then the UC channel is uncovered and the relationship between decelerations and contractions is determined. For these records a magnifying glass might help.

In the *upper panel,* the amount of spurious variability (artifact) increases late in the contraction cycle—the time period occupied by late decelerations. While many of the contractions at the beginning appear to be associated with minimal late decelerations, those at the end elicit no comparable "decelerations." It would be unusual for an otherwise healthy fetus to respond to such excessive uterine activity with such trivial, if any, decelerations. Artifact seems the better diagnosis.

In the *lower panel,* barely detectable, short-lived, "subtle" decelerations last less than 20 seconds compared to the 60 seconds of the underlying uterine contractions. In this circumstance, significant asphyxia, if any, is remote. Both of these tests prompted induction of labor but neither fetus demonstrated late decelerations during labor. The *upper panel* was obtained from a patient with a clinical diagnosis of abruptio placentae and resulted in immediate delivery of an infant who was slightly anemic at birth but survived. During the *lower panel,* the patient was febrile as a result of fever and chorioamnionitis.

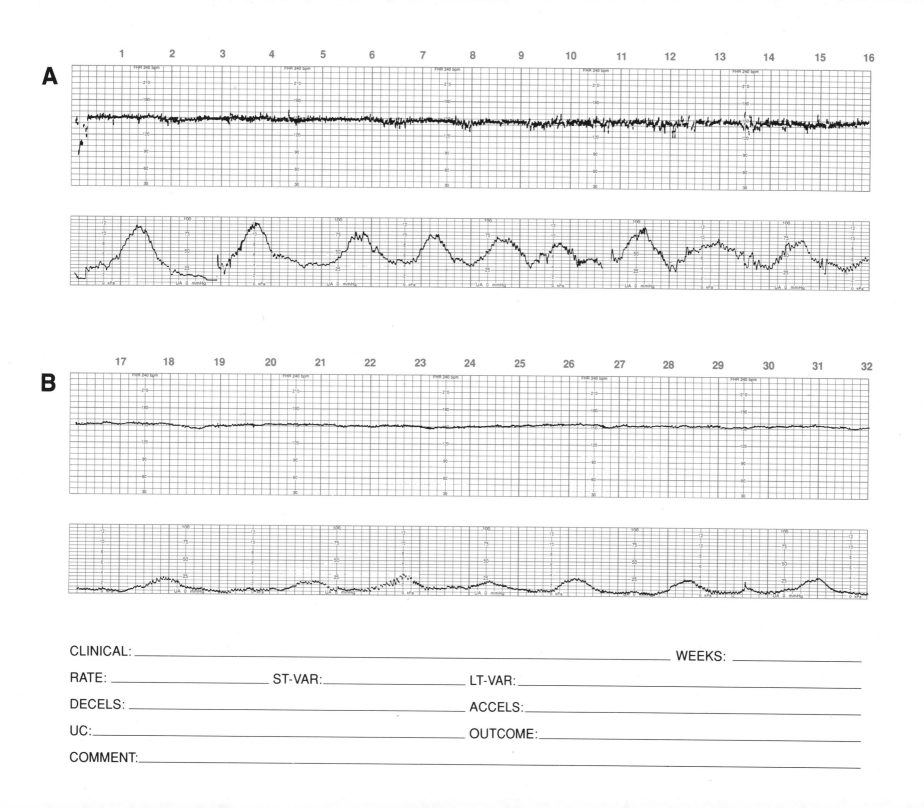

CLINICAL:_____ WEEKS:_____

RATE:_____ ST-VAR:_____ LT-VAR:_____

DECELS:_____ ACCELS:_____

UC:_____ OUTCOME:_____

COMMENT:_____

TRACING: 18

CLINICAL: Routine testing, early labor.

WEEKS: 38

RATE: 140

STV: Average.

LTV: Average.

DECELERATIONS: Absent.

ACCELERATIONS: Frequent.

UC: Early labor.

NST: Reactive.

CST: Negative.

OUTCOME: Normal.

COMMENT: This tracing illustrates the evolution of an apparent sinusoidal pattern into a clearly reactive pattern. In the *upper panel,* note the absence of decelerations, the small, but discernible effect of contractions on the heart rate pattern. The frequency of the oscillations is about 5 cpm and the amplitude about 10 bpm. While no feature of the sinusoidal pattern is diagnostic, the higher the frequency and the more irregularity in the pattern, the less likely it is to be an ominous pattern. This may represent fetal breathing or REM sleep with minimal fetal movement. Ultimately, the feature that provides the definitive commentary on this pattern is the evolution into a reactive pattern. In the *lower panel* we find frequent accelerations, some with lambda pattern (at 20M and 24M), variability, and no decelerations. This is a resilient fetus.

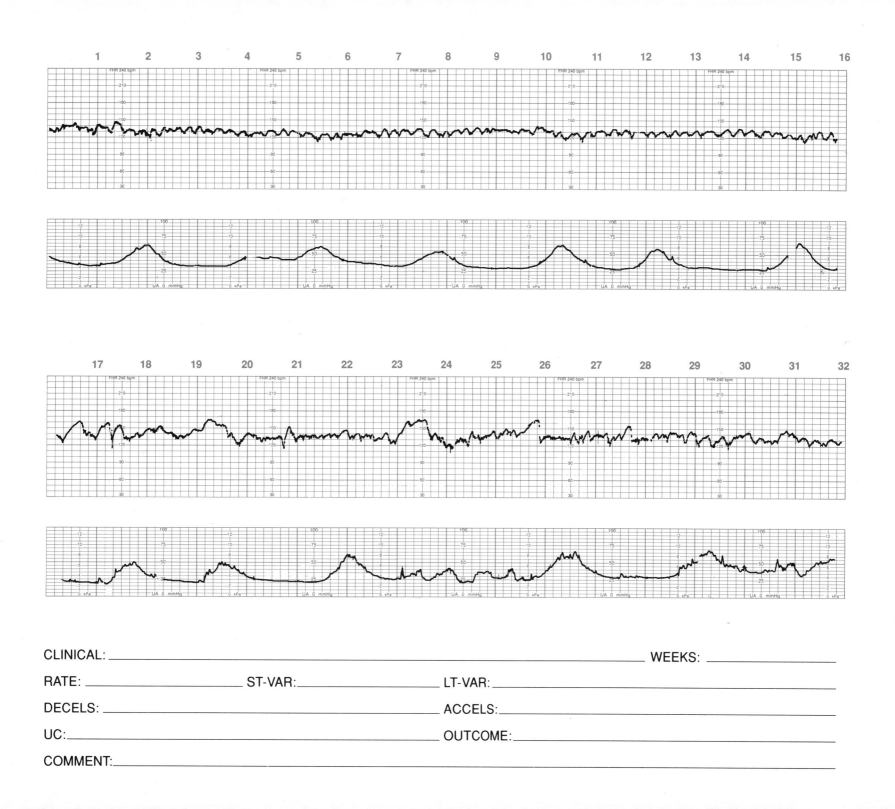

CLINICAL: _____   WEEKS: _____

RATE: _____ ST-VAR: _____   LT-VAR: _____

DECELS: _____   ACCELS: _____

UC: _____   OUTCOME: _____

COMMENT: _____

TRACING: 19

CLINICAL: Narcotic administration.

WEEKS: 38

BASELINE RATE: 150

STV: Average.

LTV: Average.

DECELERATIONS: Absent.

ACCELERATIONS: Coalesced.

UC: Irregular, high-frequency activity.

OUTCOME: Normal.

COMMENT: This tracing reveals a generally persistent, sinusoidal pattern precipitated by the maternal ingestion of cough syrup with codeine prior to this NST. The narcotized but still somewhat active fetus elicits accelerations with fetal movements at the end of the *upper panel*. This persistent type of sinusoidal pattern is often associated with either medication or certain repetitive fetal behavioral activities such as sucking or mouthing. The irregular, occasionally coupled contractions elicit no response from the fetus.

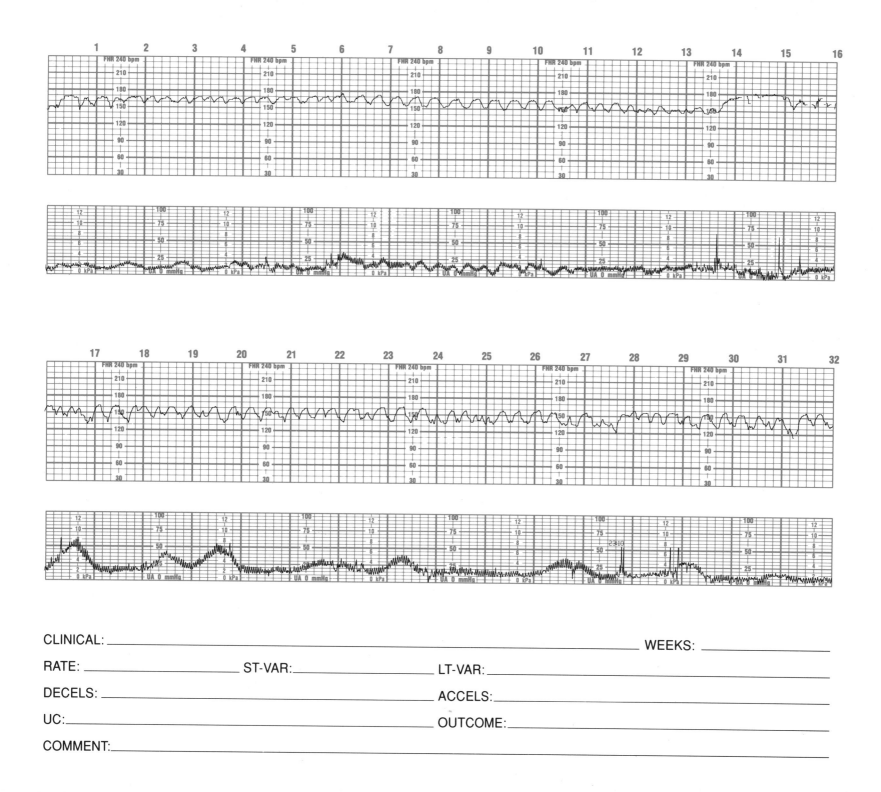

CLINICAL: _____ WEEKS: _____

RATE: _____ ST-VAR: _____ LT-VAR: _____

DECELS: _____ ACCELS: _____

UC: _____ OUTCOME: _____

COMMENT: _____

TRACING: 20

CLINICAL: Both: Early labor.

WEEKS: Both: 40

RATE: A: 120–130   B: 140

STV: A: Average. B: Absent.

LTV: Both: Average, sinusoidal.

DECELERATIONS: Both: Absent.

ACCELERATIONS: Both: Absent.

UC: Both: Oxytocin effect.

NST: Both: Nonreactive.

CST: Both: Negative.

OUTCOME: A: Normal. B: Congenital anomaly.

COMMENT: These two patterns illustrate the potential pitfalls in the interpretation of sinusoidal heart rate patterns. The *upper panel* illustrates a negative CST and a heart rate pattern which oscillates throughout most of the tracing. The first uterine contraction induces a modest deceleration, but the subsequent contractions seemingly have little impact. In addition, the oscillation frequency is fairly high (about 4–5 cpm) with some variation within the pattern. These features suggest a normal variant or breathing fetus. Indeed, this pattern will ultimately evolve into a typical reactive NST.

The *lower panel,* obtained by direct electrode in early labor, illustrates a more clear-cut sinusoidal pattern with absent short-term variability. The frequent contractions, driven by oxytocin, do not meaningfully influence the pattern. Upon delivery this fetus was found to have a congenital cardiac anomaly, a single left ventricle, and died shortly after birth. It showed no evidence of hypoxia or any neurologic abnormality. This pattern was persistent throughout the fetal tracing.

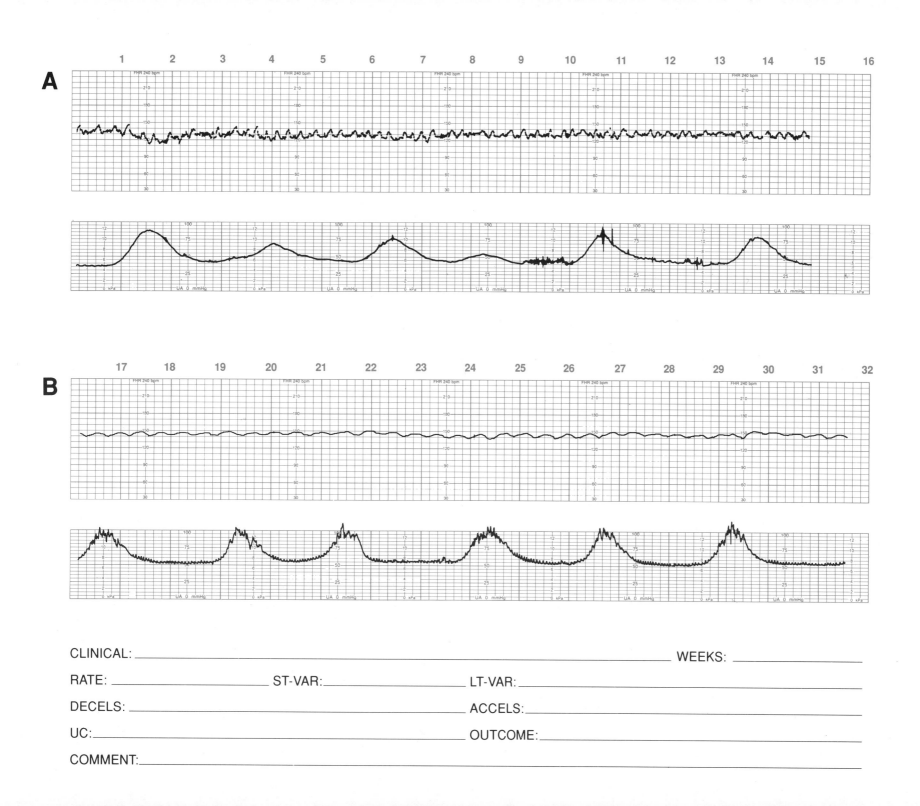

CLINICAL: _____ WEEKS: _____

RATE: _____ ST-VAR: _____ LT-VAR: _____

DECELS: _____ ACCELS: _____

UC: _____ OUTCOME: _____

COMMENT: _____

TRACING: 21

CLINICAL: Labor; fetal behavior.

WEEKS: 40

BASELINE RATE: 150

STV: Decreased.

LTV: Average, sinusoidal.

DECELERATIONS: Mild variable.

ACCELERATIONS: Absent.

UC: Labor.

OUTCOME: Fetal-neonatal anemia.

COMMENT: This tracing illustrates an intermittent sinusoidal pattern. The sinusoidal part illustrates only minimal variation and no decelerations with contractions. The variability during the nonsinusoidal part (4M to 10M) is quite flat with the suggestion of minimal late decelerations. The episode coincides with the highest frequency of uterine contractions. This sequence is quite typical of Rh isoimmunization and chronic fetal anemia. The amplitude of the sinusoidal pattern is about 10 bpm and frequency is 2–3 cpm. These wave characteristics are similar to those seen in healthy or medicated fetuses. Clues to the seriousness of the tracing are related to the fetal heart rate pattern elsewhere. If the tracing is reactive elsewhere, the most ominous sinusoidal pattern can be dismissed. If there is no normal tracing elsewhere, and the pattern alternates between nonreactivity and sinusoidal oscillations, then other abnormalities should be sought. Asphyxia is unlikely without decelerations.

Fetal anemia may be caused by fetal maternal hemorrhage, twin-to-twin transfusion, hemorrhage from obstetric abnormalities such as vasa praevia or umbilical varices, or one of many congenital anemias. Kleihauer-Betke analysis of maternal blood for fetal cells may elucidate the extent of fetal-maternal hemorrhage. These fetuses are characteristically not acidotic at the outset of labor but may become so rapidly during labor. An experienced neonatal team must be present in the delivery room to deal with any acidosis, anemia, or hypovolemia.

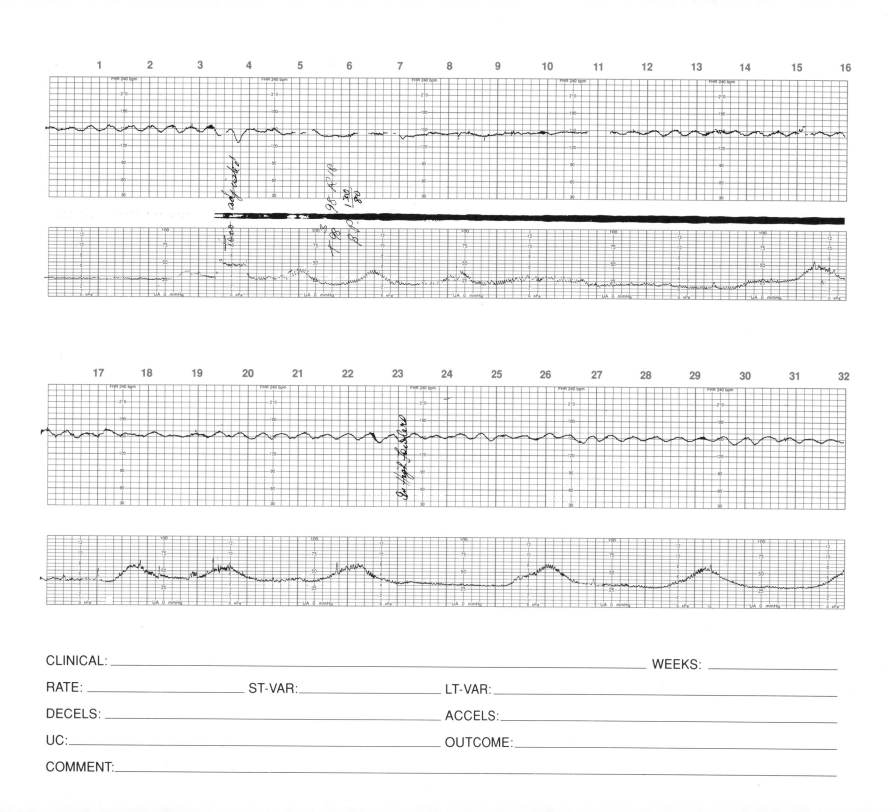

CLINICAL: _____ WEEKS: _____

RATE: _____ ST-VAR: _____ LT-VAR: _____

DECELS: _____ ACCELS: _____

UC: _____ OUTCOME: _____

COMMENT: _____

TRACING: 22

CLINICAL: Both: Uneventful prenatal course.

WEEKS: Both: 38

RATE: Both: 150–160

STV: A: Decreased.   B: Average.

LTV: Both: Average to increased.

DECELS: Both: Variable.

ACCELS: Both: Variable ("shoulders").

UC: A: Irregular, coupling. B: Second stage

OUTCOME: Both: Apgar scores, 8/9; uneventful neonatal course.

COMMENT: The *upper panel* reveals a sinusoidal FHR pattern associated with narcotic administration in a particularly susceptible fetus. The sine wave is characteristically 2–6 cpm, 5–15 bpm in amplitude, and will wax and wane only minimally. Note the occasional variable decelerations, with contractions that modulate only slightly the sinusoidal pattern. There is considerable irregularity within the cycles of the sine wave. The preceding tracing was quite reassuring. Implicitly, this tracing again illustrates the benefit of a baseline tracing prior to administration of any medication to the mother or fetus.

The *lower panel* illustrates larger oscillatory excursions that are sometimes confused with the sinusoidal pattern. These dramatic excursions that occur at the end of variable decelerations are sometimes referred to as saltatory (jumping) or "vagal" patterns. Such changes are seen in resilient (unmedicated) fetuses, and rarely deteriorate. This infant was born with the cord wrapped twice around the neck.

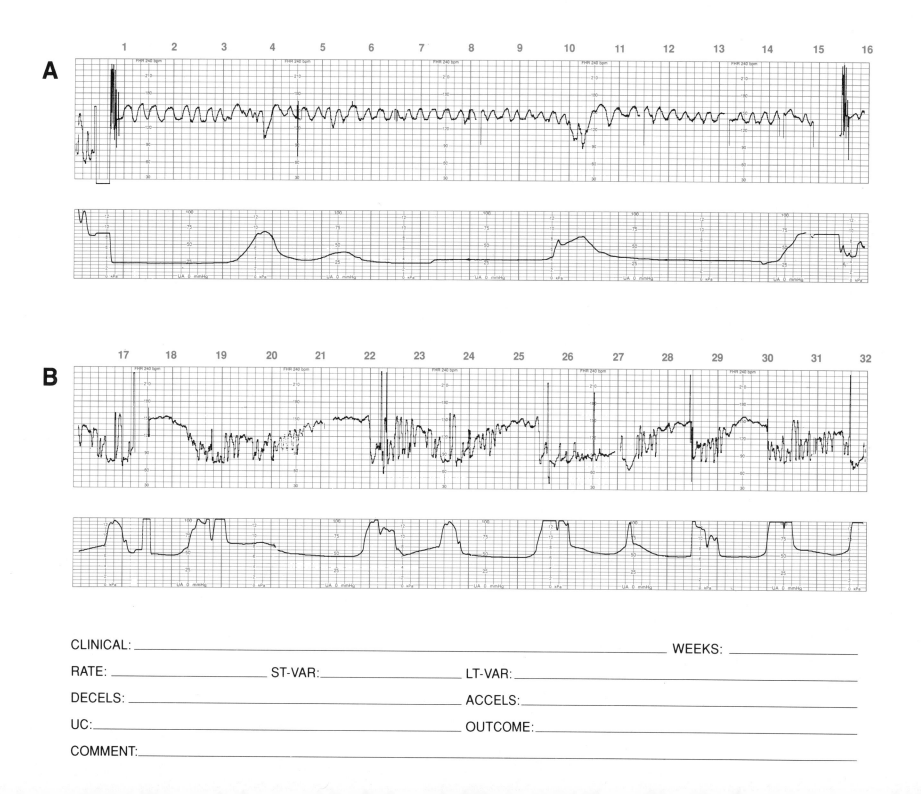

CLINICAL: _____ WEEKS: _____

RATE: _____ ST-VAR: _____ LT-VAR: _____

DECELS: _____ ACCELS: _____

UC:_____ OUTCOME: _____

COMMENT:_____

TRACING: 23

CLINICAL: Hydramnios.

WEEKS: 39

RATE: 140–150

STV: Decreased.

LTV: Average.

DECELERATIONS: Prolonged.

ACCELERATIONS: Absent.

UC: Irregular, coupled.

NST: Nonreactive.

CST: Negative.

OUTCOME: Maternal-fetal transfusion; infant survived.

COMMENT: This interesting tracing of a moderately anemic fetus underscores the limitations of predicating intervention solely on the basis of the sinusoidal pattern. In this fetus, two alternating patterns emerge. One pattern associated with a baseline of 140–150 bpm contains minimal short-term variability and, from 21M onward, a sinusoidal pattern. The other pattern, at about 130 bpm, seems to show greater short-term variability. The epochs evolve smoothly into one another during a contraction, but their duration is unpredictable. It is inappropriate to consider these changes as indicative of decelerations. They bear no consistent length or relationship to uterine contractions. The irregular contractions, which occasionally couple, do not provoke decelerations.

How to explain these epochs? They might represent fetal breathing movements, a discordant pattern of a pair of fetuses, or counting of the maternal rate. The issue was never resolved except that only a single fetus was delivered, and the maternal rate during the tracing was about 80 bpm.

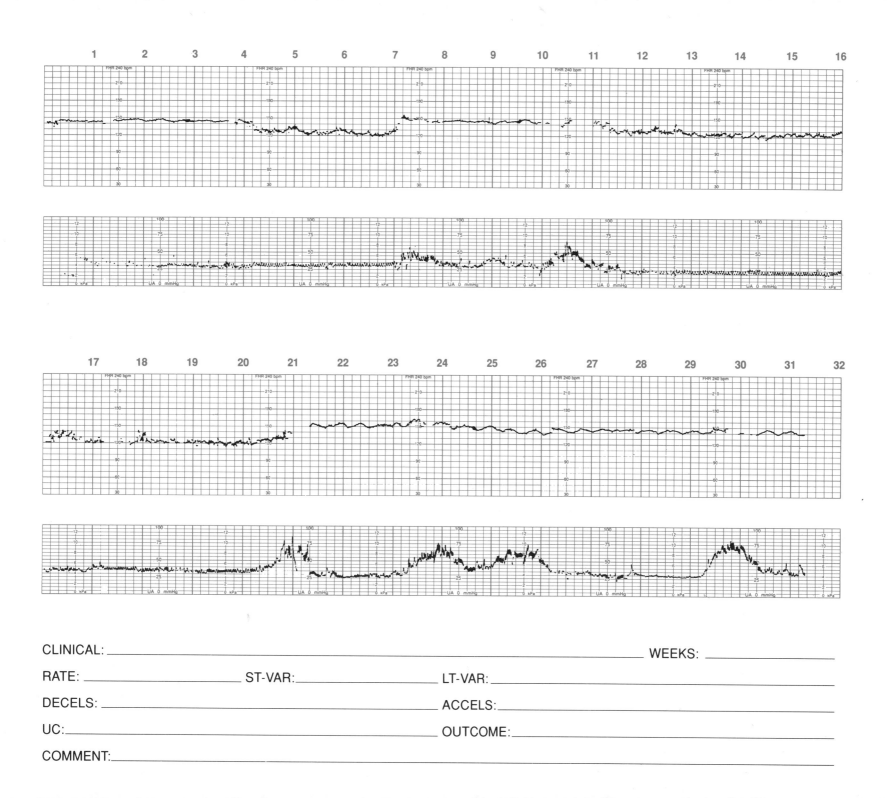

CLINICAL: _____ WEEKS: _____

RATE: _____ ST-VAR: _____ LT-VAR: _____

DECELS: _____ ACCELS: _____

UC:_____ OUTCOME:_____

COMMENT:_____

TRACING: 24

CLINICAL: Labor.

WEEKS: 40

BASELINE RATE: 160

STV: Average.

LTV: Increased.

DECELERATIONS: Variable, prolonged.

ACCELERATIONS: Small.

UC: Coupling, oxytocin.

OUTCOME: Normal.

COMMENT: This tracing begins with an elevated baseline rate of 160 bpm and abrupt, rather regularly spaced, small vertical spikes. These changes are consistent with a transient fetal arrhythmia (not documented). Beginning at 5M the variability increases and late-appearing decelerations begin which are probably better characterized as variable decelerations. There are variable decelerations with several of the reasonably spaced contractions, but the baseline rate and average variability are maintained. At 18M, in response to the coupling of contractions, a prolonged deceleration appears. At 22M, as the rate attempts to recover, the variability becomes saltatory (increased), reflecting cardiac compensation after the insult. The baseline then rises to a rate higher than the previous rate for several minutes until returning to the previous rate of 160 bpm. This process of deceleration and recovery may continue throughout labor and present neither indication for intervention nor evidence of asphyxia or injury as long as the heart tones always return to the previous rate and pattern within a reasonable period of time (e.g., 20 minutes).

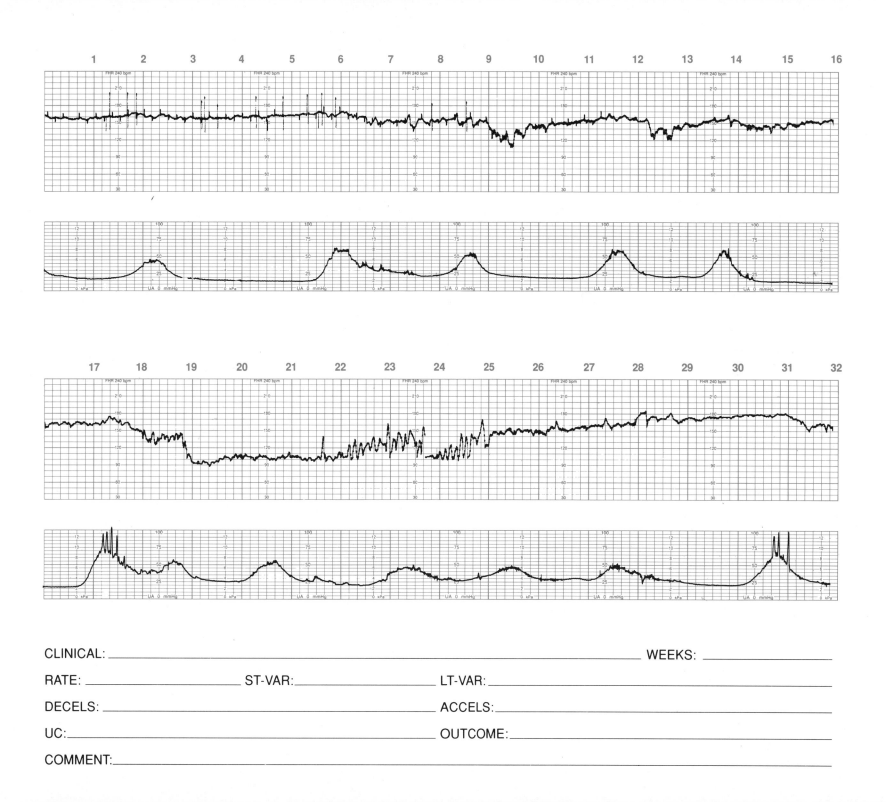

CLINICAL: _____ WEEKS: _____

RATE: _____ ST-VAR: _____ LT-VAR: _____

DECELS: _____ ACCELS: _____

UC: _____ OUTCOME: _____

COMMENT: _____

TRACING: 25

CLINICAL: Second-stage labor.

WEEKS: 39

BASELINE RATE: 170

STV: Average.

LTV: Increased.

DECELERATIONS: Variable.

ACCELERATIONS: Absent.

UC: Bearing down, breathing.

OUTCOME: Apgar scores 9/9; normal infant.

COMMENT: This tracing illustrates the presumed effects of fetal head compression during the second stage of labor. The elevated baseline rate and decreased baseline variability are punctuated by recurrent decelerations which for the most part are confined to the time period during contractions. Whether these are called variable decelerations or early decelerations is of little consequence. Note that the decelerations tend to be proportional in amplitude and duration to the underlying uterine contractions and that the excursions within the decelerations tend to correspond to the alternating efforts at expulsion and relaxation during the contraction. The variability during the deceleration increases as a result. At 15M, coinciding with a change in position and coupling of the contraction, the deceleration is prolonged but recovers promptly. With the patient on her back the very frequent contractions induce decelerations associated with above-average variability. The deceleration at 27M lasts well beyond the contraction and recovers to a higher rate thereafter. This rise in baseline variability and perhaps some slowing of the baseline rate associated with compulsive pushing in the second stage appear harmless enough, but doubtless represent considerable autonomic interaction, the result of the elevated intracranial pressure and fetal hypertension necessary to maintain perfusion in the head. Very rarely this may lead to disaster (see tracing 84).

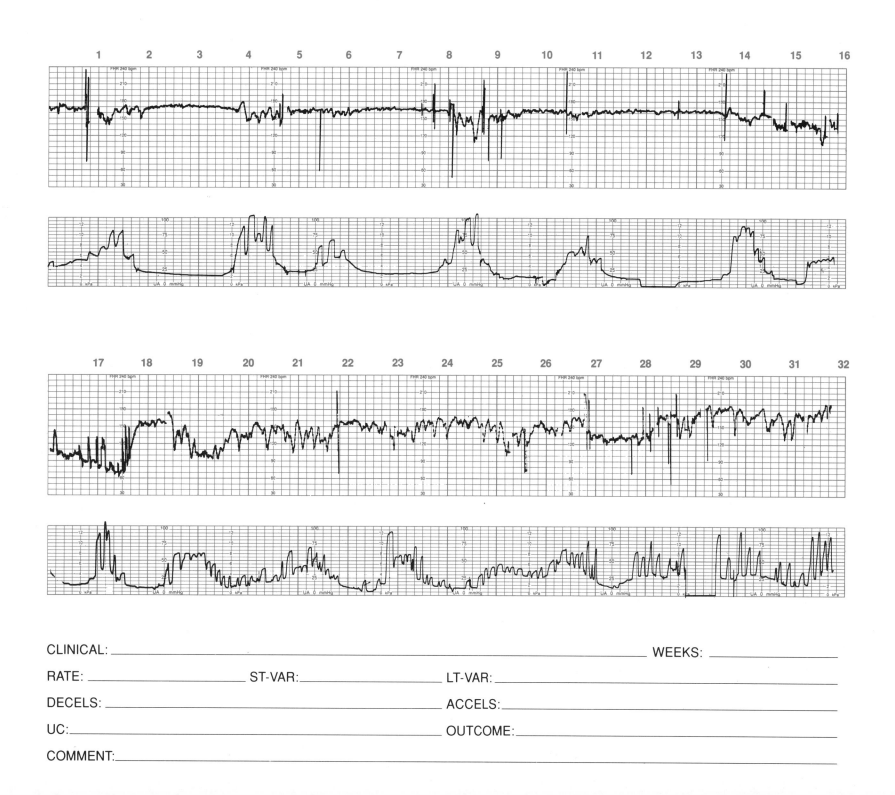

CLINICAL: _____ WEEKS: _____

RATE: _____ ST-VAR: _____ LT-VAR: _____

DECELS: _____ ACCELS: _____

UC: _____ OUTCOME: _____

COMMENT: _____

TRACING: 26

CLINICAL: Both: Hypertension.

WEEKS: 39

RATE: 120

STV: A: Average. B: Decreased.

LTV: A: Average. B: Decreased.

DECELERATIONS: A: Absent. B: Prolonged.

ACCELERATIONS: A: Sporadic, coalesced. B: Absent.

UC: Both: Excessive.

NST: A: Reactive. B: Nonreactive.

CST: A: Negative. B: Equivocal.

OUTCOME: Both: Normal.

COMMENT: This tracing presents the varied responses to uterine hyperstimulation. In the *upper panel* an obviously reactive baby encounters sustained uterine hypertonus lasting more than 5 minutes. Note the abundant fetal movement in anticipation of the hypertonus. The movement continues throughout the first several minutes of uterine hypertonus associated with accelerations in the fetal heart rate. As the movements decrease, then cease, so do the accelerations in the heart rate. Despite the prolonged hypertonus, there are no decelerations. Nor is there any rise in the baseline rate. At the end of the panel fetal movements resume with the appearance of accelerations.

In the *lower panel,* spontaneous uterine hypertonus lasting about 10 minutes provokes a prolonged deceleration and the suggestion of a late deceleration during recovery at 26M. This pattern evolved into a transient tachycardia with absent variability, then returned to its previous reactive pattern.

In the *upper panel* the hypertonus was related to the administration of oxytocin. In the *lower panel* it was spontaneous. About 2% of tracings will manifest spontaneous hypertonus although few as dramatic as that presented in the *lower panel.* About 50% of the time uterine hypertonus induces prolonged decelerations that for the most part are inconsequential. In each of these cases, obvious reactivity resumed immediately. Ultrasound scanning showed normal amniotic fluid volume and no intervention was undertaken in either case.

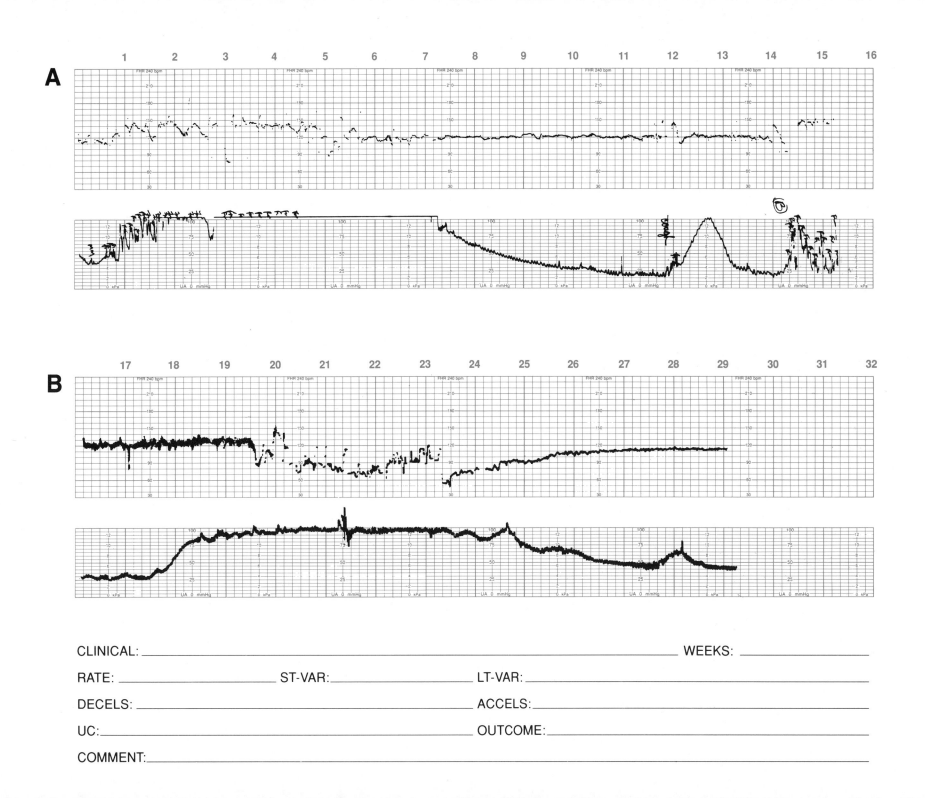

CLINICAL: _____ WEEKS: _____

RATE: _____ ST-VAR:_____ LT-VAR: _____

DECELS: _____ ACCELS:_____

UC:_____ OUTCOME:_____

COMMENT:_____

TRACING: 27

CLINICAL: Maternal cocaine use.

WEEKS: 37

BASELINE RATE: 120

STV: Average.

LTV: Exaggerated.

DECELERATIONS: Occasional variable.

ACCELERATIONS: Isolated; shoulders.

UC: Early labor, irregular.

OUTCOME: Normal.

COMMENT: This tracing reflects exaggerated variability (saltatory pattern) consistent with neurologic overstimulation of the fetus as may be seen in unmedicated labor. Note the irregular maternal breathing. There are obvious accelerations and exaggerated variability throughout. There are also mild to moderate variable decelerations, probably reflecting decreased amniotic fluid. At this point the fetus is well oxygenated but simply demonstrating autonomic arousal. This fetus is reactive in every respect, though it does not show the usual pattern of rest/activity cycles.

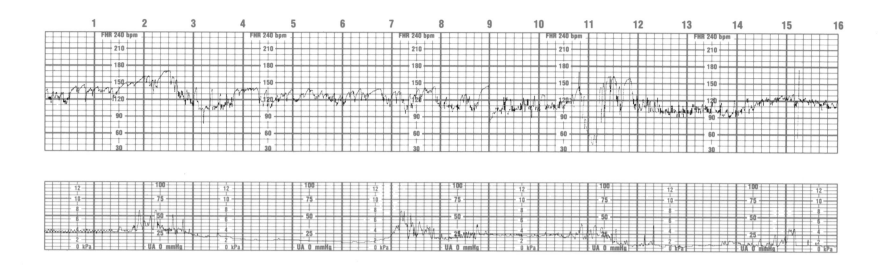

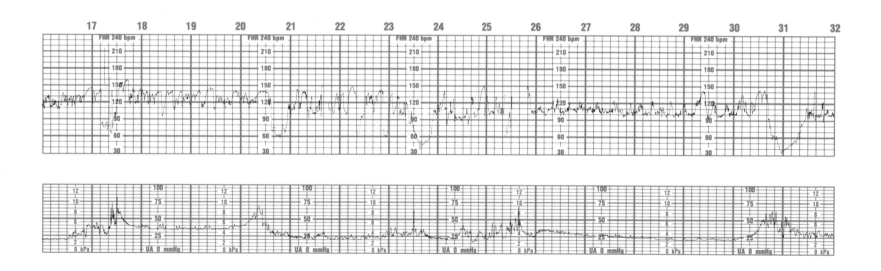

CLINICAL: _____ WEEKS: _____

RATE: _____ ST-VAR: _____ LT-VAR: _____

DECELS: _____ ACCELS: _____

UC: _____ OUTCOME: _____

COMMENT: _____

TRACING: 28

CLINICAL: A: Routine. B: Decreased fetal movement.

WEEKS: 41

RATE: A: 140   B: 110

STV: A: Average. B: Decreased.

LTV: A: Average. B: Decreased.

DECELERATIONS: Both: Variable.

ACCELERATIONS: A: Sporadic, shoulders. B: Absent.

UC: A: Irregular. B: Early labor.

NST: A: Reactive. B: Nonreactive.

CST: A: Negative. B: Positive.

OUTCOME: A: Normal. B: Neonatal death.
Both: Meconium stained.

COMMENT: The *upper panel* reveals variable decelerations in association with reactivity. The variable decelerations are introduced by accelerations (shoulders) and are followed by similar accelerations. This frequent association of variable decelerations with fetal movement presumably arises when fetal movement causes some cord entanglement and precipitates variable decelerations unrelated to any compromise. This sequence tends to develop under conditions of oligohydramnios, and perhaps with a nuchal cord. Shortly after this tracing the infant was delivered in satisfactory condition.

The *lower panel* is remarkably different. Here the fetus reveals no accelerations and isolated, apparently early, decelerations. Early decelerations are extraordinarily unusual in antepartum testing and almost invariably evolve into more typical variable decelerations. The combination of variable decelerations and nonreactive pattern is a potentially ominous combination which deserves immediate attention, evaluation, and likely early delivery. The potential for chronic compromise with such tracings is significant.

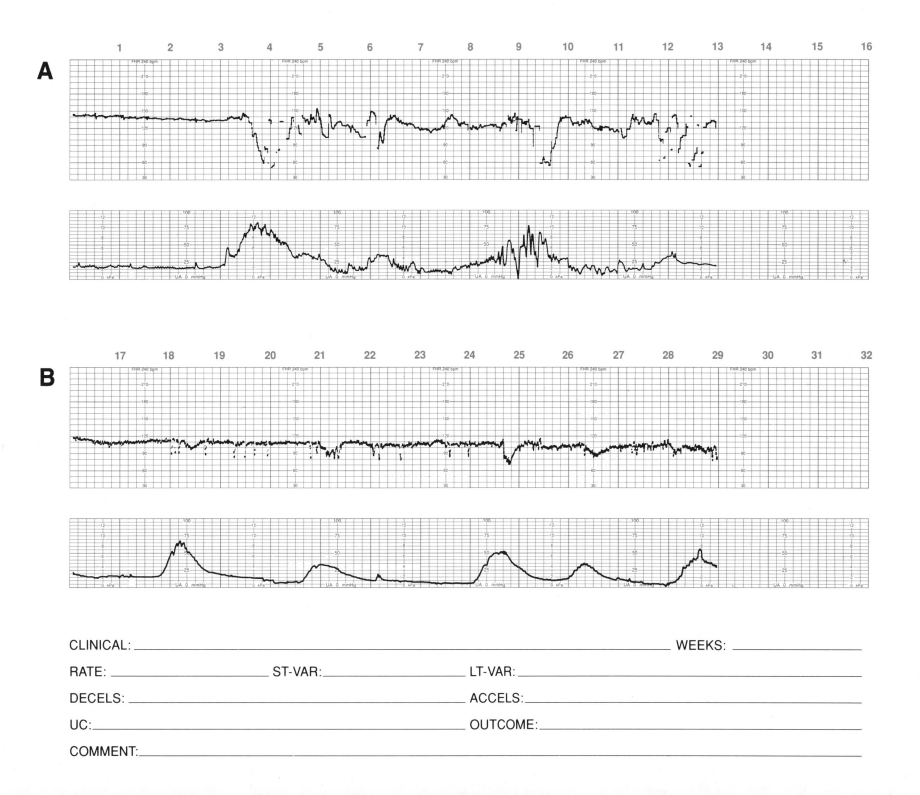

CLINICAL:_____ WEEKS:_____

RATE:_____ ST-VAR:_____ LT-VAR:_____

DECELS:_____ ACCELS:_____

UC:_____ OUTCOME:_____

COMMENT:_____

TRACING: 29

CLINICAL: Postdate pregnancy, early labor, oligohydramnios.

WEEKS: 43

RATE: 120

STV: Average, increased.

LTV: Average.

DECELERATIONS: Prolonged, variable.

ACCELERATIONS: Variable.

UC: Irregular.

OUTCOME: Meconium-stained; postmaturity syndrome; normal outcome.

COMMENT: This pattern, obtained in a postdate pregnancy, reveals a low baseline rate, normal to increased variability, and both broad and shallow decelerations. The decelerations should not be classified as late; they vary considerably in duration, amplitude, and relationship to the underlying contraction. The baseline shows no tendency toward tachycardia. While these features tend to deny a fetal indication for intervention, more decelerations should be expected later in labor. These findings, present during antepartum testing in the term or postdate fetus, are now considered sufficient indication for termination of pregnancy by induction of labor.

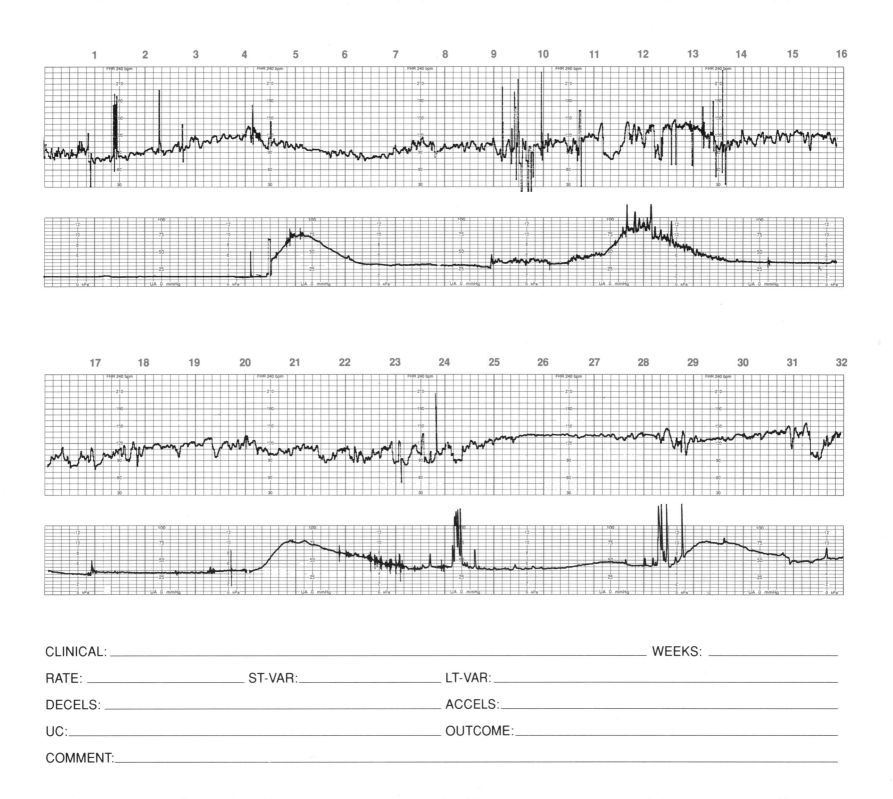

CLINICAL: _____   WEEKS: _____

RATE: _____   ST-VAR: _____   LT-VAR: _____

DECELS: _____   ACCELS: _____

UC: _____   OUTCOME: _____

COMMENT: _____

TRACING: 30

CLINICAL: A: Postdate. B: Routine.

WEEKS: 42

RATE: Both: 130

STV: A: Decreased. B: Average.

LTV: A: Decreased. B: Average.

DECELERATIONS: A: Prolonged. B: Absent.

ACCELERATIONS: A: Occasional sporadic B: Numerous.

UC: Both: Infrequent.

NST: A: Nonreactive. B: Reactive.

CST: A: Equivocal. B: Negative.

OUTCOME: A: Postmature. B: Normal.

COMMENT: The *upper panel* illustrates a single prolonged deceleration without similar decelerations with adjacent uterine contractions. This feature alone precludes the diagnosis of late decelerations, however abnormal the test. Note the two episodes of double counting during the deceleration just before and just after 5M. These decelerations may reflect either umbilical cord compression or, remotely, fetal breathing movements. The reactivity at the very beginning of this panel and the failure of the deceleration to repeat with a subsequent contraction suggest that whatever it is, it is transient and recoverable. Ultrasound investi-gation of amniotic fluid volume ought to be carried out and if the baby is at term then intervention should be considered.

The *lower panel* illustrates the potential pitfalls of both the lambda pattern and the importance of defining a baseline. In this instance, abundant, coalesced accelerations accompany fetal movements. The temptation to refer to them as decelerations between 18M and 20M and between 26M and 29M should be avoided in that they show no consistent relationship to the uterine contractions. If anything, they begin concurrently with the onset of the contraction. This is a reassuring tracing.

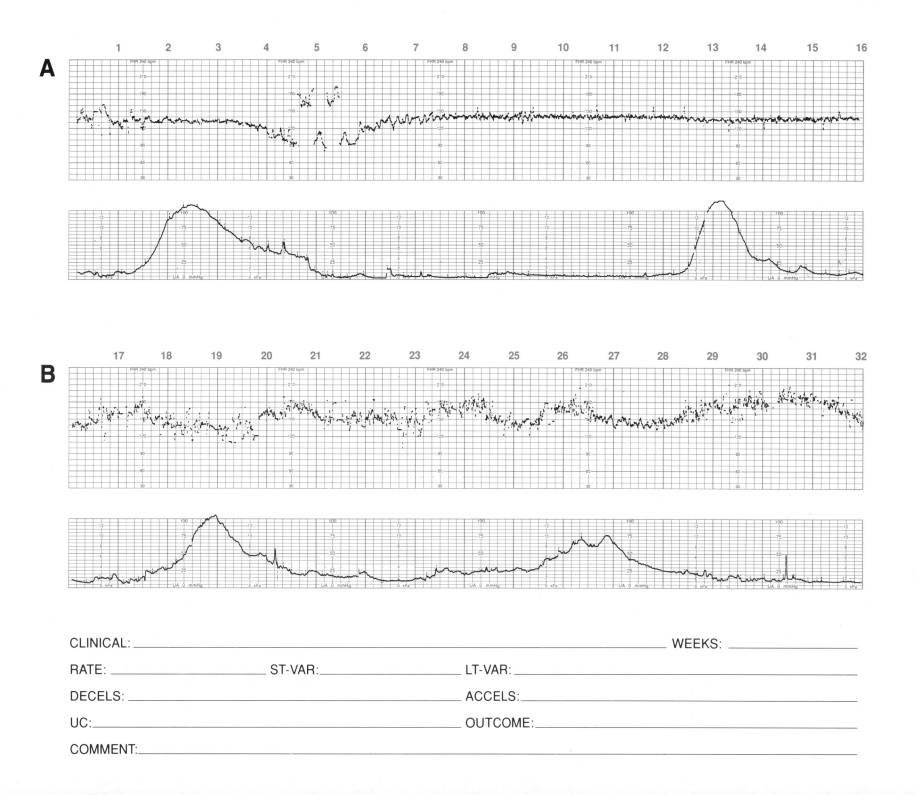

CLINICAL: _____ WEEKS: _____

RATE: _____ ST-VAR: _____ LT-VAR: _____

DECELS: _____ ACCELS: _____

UC: _____ OUTCOME: _____

COMMENT: _____

TRACING: 31

CLINICAL: Premature rupture of the membranes; febrile mother.

WEEKS: 36

RATE: 180–190

STV: Decreased.

LTV: Decreased.

DECELERATIONS: Variable!

ACCELERATIONS: Absent.

UC: Upper: Irregular. oxytocin.

NST: Nonreactive.

CST: Equivocal.

OUTCOME: Apgar scores 3/6; neonatal sepsis.

COMMENT: This tracing illustrates the potential confusion in the evaluation of decelerations during antepartum testing. Note the characteristic features of oxytocin stimulation, especially on the *lower panel*. Here the contractions are relatively constant in amplitude and appearance and, to some extent, interval. Spontaneous contractions tend to be far more variable in amplitude, duration, and interval.

The tracing reveals baseline tachycardia and diminished variability, more obvious in the *lower panel*. Decelerations appear with several of the contractions on the *upper panel* and virtually all of the contractions on the *lower panel*. They are either unrelated to the contraction (1M), within the contraction (6M), or follow the contraction (at 11M and 13M). In addition, they do not maintain any obvious proportionality to the amplitude of the underlying uterine contraction.

In the *lower panel* the decelerations, though consistent with each contraction, tend to show an inconsistent onset in relation to the contraction. While calling them late decelerations is understandable, the most reasonable designation is variable decelerations. Irrespective of the designation of the decelerations, the combination of decelerations, tachycardia, minimal reactivity, and diminished baseline variability is of great concern and should prompt intervention.

This pattern was obtained in a patient at 36 weeks' gestation with premature rupture of the membranes and chorioamnionitis. At delivery, the infant had Apgar scores of 3 and 6, and though infected, revealed no significant acidosis.

Fever in the mother increases both fetal and placental oxygen requirements. It elevates both maternal and fetal heart rates, and may induce late decelerations of modest amplitude. Overt deterioration of the fetus as a result of moderate maternal fever develops rarely, if at all. Prolonged, unattended high fever or infection may cause fetal deterioration and death.

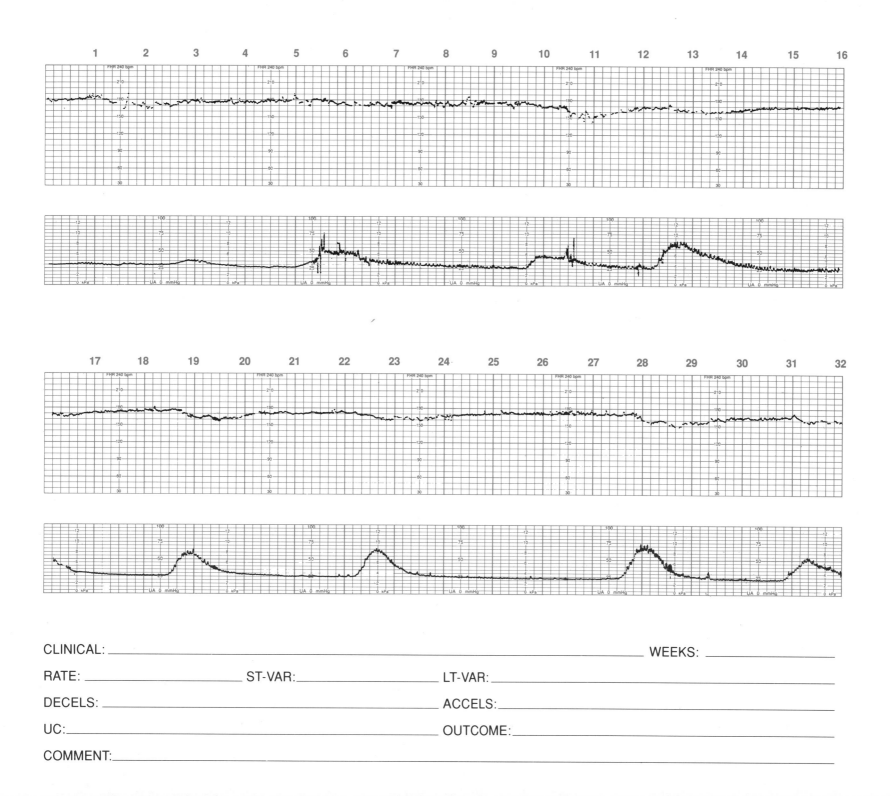

CLINICAL:_____ WEEKS:_____

RATE:_____ ST-VAR:_____ LT-VAR:_____

DECELS:_____ ACCELS:_____

UC:_____ OUTCOME:_____

COMMENT:_____

TRACING: 32

CLINICAL: Postdate pregnancy.

WEEKS: 42

RATE: A: 160–170   B: 140–150

STV: Average to increased.

LTV: Average to increased.

DECELERATIONS: Prolonged.

ACCELERATIONS: Occasional sporadic.

UC: Occasional.

NST: Probably reactive.

CST: Equivocal.

OUTCOME: Postmature infant; intact survival.

COMMENT: These tracings, obtained an hour apart from the same fetus, reveal several characteristic FHR features of the postdate fetus. These features include decelerations that do not subscribe to any obvious pattern. They are shallow, of variable duration, and show exaggerated variability during the deceleration. The baseline shows average to increased variability and some accelerations, more obvious in the *lower panel*. The elevated heart rate and the decelerations suggest that this postdate fetus is at increased risk of meconium passage and oligohydramnios and fetal wasting (dysmaturity). Nevertheless, there is no evidence of diminished oxygen transport. The infant, meconium-stained and obviously wasted, thrived.

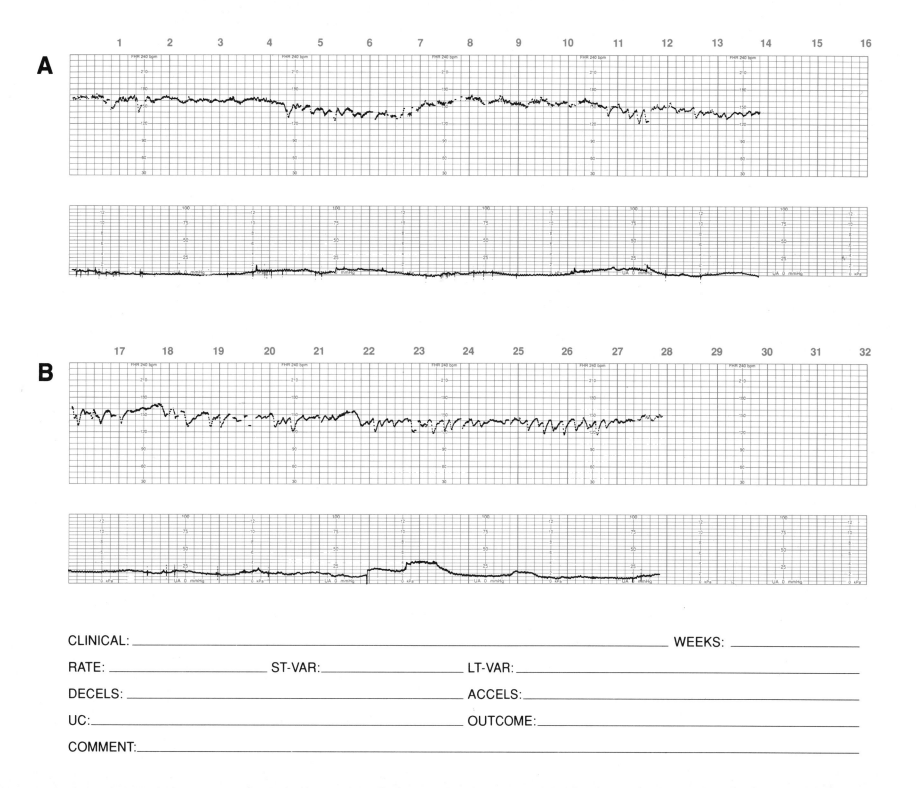

CLINICAL: _____ WEEKS: _____

RATE: _____ ST-VAR:_____ LT-VAR: _____

DECELS: _____ ACCELS:_____

UC:_____ OUTCOME:_____

COMMENT:_____

TRACING: 33

CLINICAL: Hypertension.

WEEKS: 38

RATE: 140

STV: Average.

LTV: Decreased.

DECELERATIONS: Probably variable.

ACCELERATIONS: Minimal.

UC: Regular toward end.

NST: Nonreactive.

CST: Suspicious.

OUTCOME: Normal.

COMMENT: This tracing illustrates minimal reactivity and a number of decelerations. The *upper panel* is introduced with a variable deceleration, probably associated with either fetal movement, abdominal manipulation, or perhaps even a pelvic examination. Despite the considerable artifact associated with this apparent deceleration, it is introduced and followed by small accelerations (shoulders). Between 6M and 7M a small deceleration (possibly artifact) seems to be preceded by fetal movement (the spike on the UC channel) and a small acceleration. Low amplitude decelerations (possibly late decelerations) accompany the last 2 contractions on the *upper panel*.

On the *lower panel,* the regular amplitude and interval of the contractions suggest oxytocin effect. Here, each of the contractions is associated with obvious decelerations that seem to extend into the next contraction. These decelerations are longer and seemingly out of proportion to the length of the underlying contractions. In addition, one can infer variability at the base of the decelerations. The baseline rate remains stable and an acceleration accompanies fetal movement at about 24M. Although there is great temptation to call this a positive CST, this likely represents either fetal breathing or the decelerations associated with oligohydramnios. On the basis of the test, the patient was induced and found to have recurrent variable decelerations but a normal outcome.

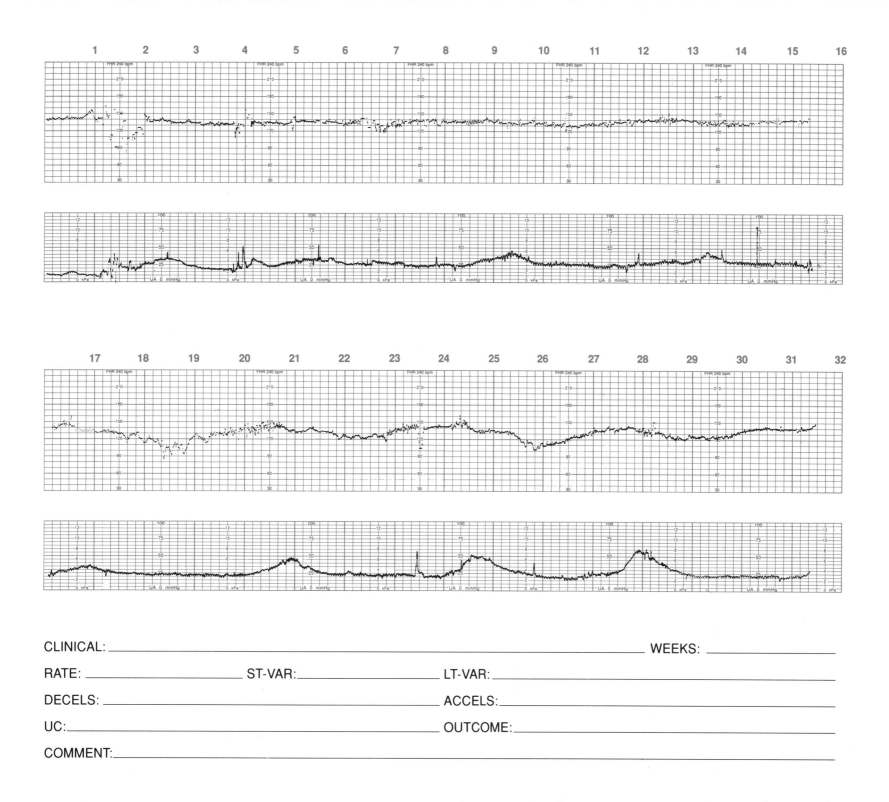

CLINICAL: _____ WEEKS: _____

RATE: _____ ST-VAR: _____ LT-VAR: _____

DECELS: _____ ACCELS: _____

UC: _____ OUTCOME: _____

COMMENT: _____

TRACING: 34

CLINICAL: Pregnancy-induced hypertension.

WEEKS: 38

RATE: 140

STV: Decreased.

LTV: Decreased.

DECELERATIONS: Late.

ACCELERATIONS: Absent.

UC: Occasional.

NST: Nonreactive.

CST: Equivocal.

OUTCOME: Apgar scores 2/5; ultimately normal outcome.

COMMENT: This tracing illustrates the problem of correctly identifying decelerations. This nonreactive NST also contains intermittent, late-appearing decelerations. These decelerations do not recur with consecutive contractions of similar amplitude. Thus, the tracing does not fulfill the criteria for either a positive or negative CST and, if not carried further, would be classified as an equivocal CST. These decelerations are unlikely to represent fetal compromise in that they occur with smaller contractions (10M and perhaps 29M) but are absent with the larger contraction. It is axiomatic that external tocotransducers do not allow quantitation of the intrauterine pressure.

But if the tocotransducer is not moved, the belt not tightened, and the patient's position not changed, then it is reasonable to infer the relative strength of the contractions from the external tracing. The most likely explanation is that of fetal breathing, but this was never confirmed. The absence of reactivity may be explained on the basis of maternal ingestion of phenobarbital.

On the basis of the nonreactive NST and equivocal CST in the near-term fetus, intervention was undertaken. The infant was somewhat depressed at birth but the umbilical cord gases were normal.

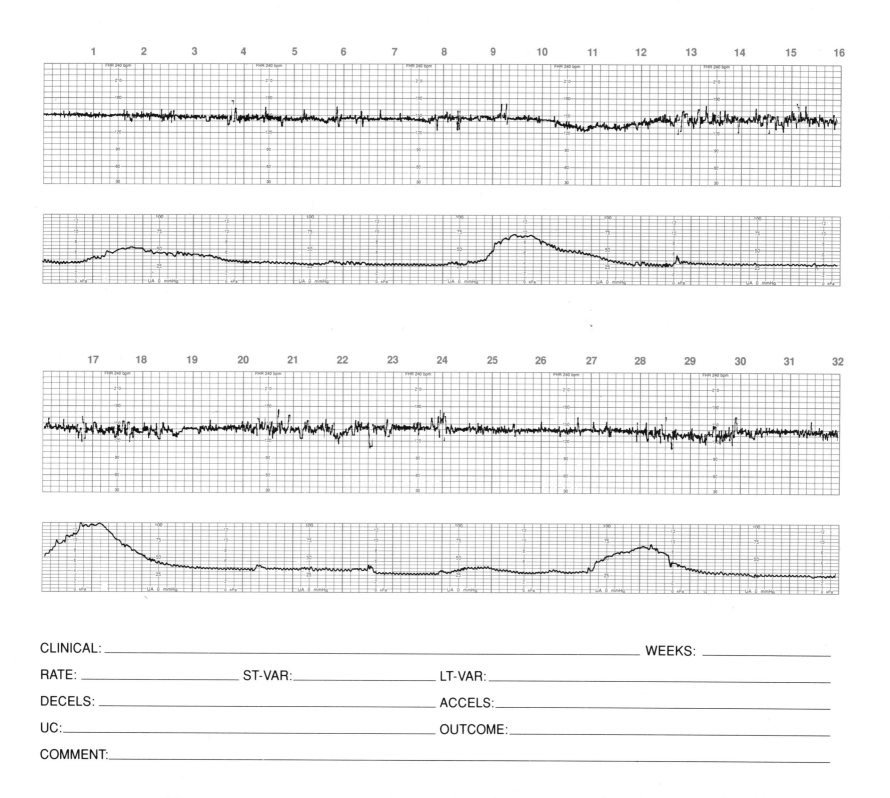

CLINICAL: _____ WEEKS: _____

RATE: _____ ST-VAR: _____ LT-VAR: _____

DECELS: _____ ACCELS: _____

UC: _____ OUTCOME: _____

COMMENT: _____

TRACING: 35

CLINICAL: Postdate pregnancy.

WEEKS: 41

BASELINE RATE: 145

STV: Decreased.

LTV: Decreased.

DECELERATIONS: "Late."

ACCELERATIONS: Absent.

UC: Oxytocin effect.

OUTCOME: Cesarean section; Apgar scores 2/7.

COMMENT: This tracing reveals late decelerations and decreased variability during an early latent phase of labor. The decelerations later resolve and do not reappear, even during oxytocin induction. The most obvious explanation is not asphyxia but fetal breathing! Note that the variability is maintained and that there is no apparent compensatory rise in the heart rate as a result of this sequence of "late" decelerations. The clue lies in the appearance of the high frequency oscillations on the UC channel which appear when the patient is turned on her back at 10M. These represent fetal breathing and not maternal respirations.

The absence of decelerations despite the greater amount of uterine activity in the *lower panel* again indicates the fetus is not asphyxiated.

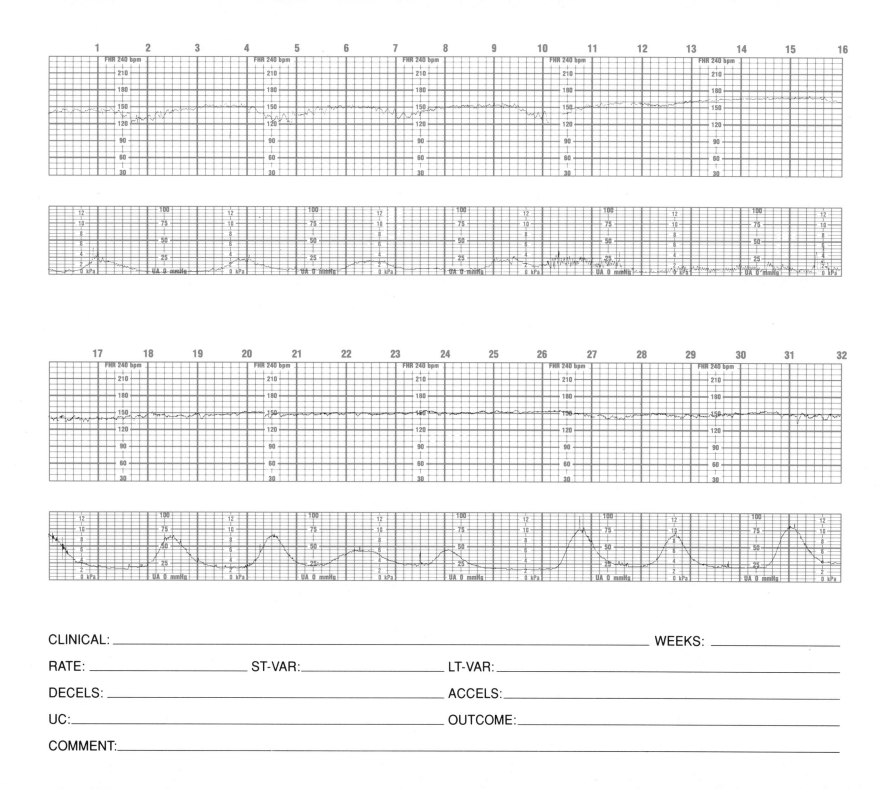

CLINICAL: _____ WEEKS: _____

RATE: _____ ST-VAR: _____ LT-VAR: _____

DECELS: _____ ACCELS: _____

UC: _____ OUTCOME: _____

COMMENT: _____

TRACING: 36

CLINICAL: Maternal diabetes.

WEEKS: 37

RATE: 150

STV: Average to increased.

LTV: Average to increased.

DECELERATIONS: Not late.

ACCELERATIONS: Absent.

UC: Regular; FBM.

NST: Nonreactive.

CST: Equivocal.

OUTCOME: Normal outcome; resilient fetus.

COMMENT: This interesting tracing, obtained with abdominal ECG electrodes, invites classification as a positive CST. The *upper* panel contains unequivocal decelerations that appear late in timing, but there is significant variation in the onset and duration of the decelerations. The baseline variability is average and shows no tendency to tachycardia or decreased variability. The UC channel reveals high frequency, low amplitude, somewhat irregular spikes which represent fetal breathing movements. Note that when the fetal breathing movements cease between 16M and 20M, the decelerations also disappear.

The outcome of this baby was normal and the test, originally called a positive CST, was ultimately classified as false-positive. The appearance of FBM, best determined by real-time ultrasound, appears to be a sign of well-being. FBM may be seen on the UC channel if attention is paid to the application of the toco-transducer. Instead of applying the transducer over the center of the uterine fundus, placing it over a palpable extremity or shoulder will increase the likelihood of detecting FBM.

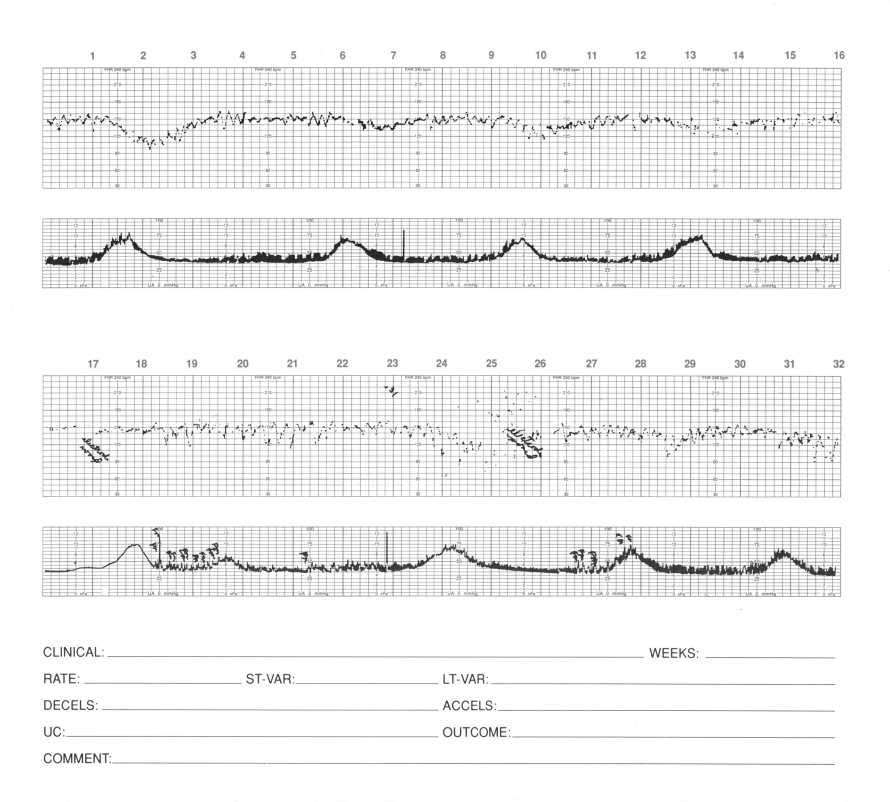

CLINICAL: _____ WEEKS: _____

RATE: _____ ST-VAR: _____ LT-VAR: _____

DECELS: _____ ACCELS: _____

UC: _____ OUTCOME: _____

COMMENT: _____

TRACING: 37

CLINICAL: Uneventful prenatal course.

WEEKS: 39

BASELINE RATE: 150

STV: Average.

LTV: Average.

DECELERATIONS: Late.

ACCELERATIONS: None.

UC: Regular; effect of epidural.

OUTCOME: Apgar scores 9/9; uneventful neonatal course.

COMMENT: This tracing illustrates the development of late decelerations following epidural anesthesia and maternal hypotension. In this previously reassuring tracing, one can easily follow the evolution and resolution of the late decelerations. It is often difficult, however, even in retrospect, to decide on the first late deceleration in a series. Is the deviation at 6M a late deceleration? Often, not-so-definitive late decelerations become recognizable only when subsequent, more characteristic features appear. Note the increased frequency of contractions immediately after the epidural. During recovery, there is a rise in the baseline and a diminution in the baseline variability along with some decrease in the frequency of contractions. The decelerations should be managed by the administration of oxygen, lateral positioning, hydration, and diminution of oxytocin (if running). At the same time, it is reasonable to presume that in this previously normal fetus, these maneuvers will indeed correct the transient, doubtless inconsequential, episode of distress. Prehydration and maintenance of the patient in the lateral position after the anesthesia will dramatically reduce the incidence of late decelerations.

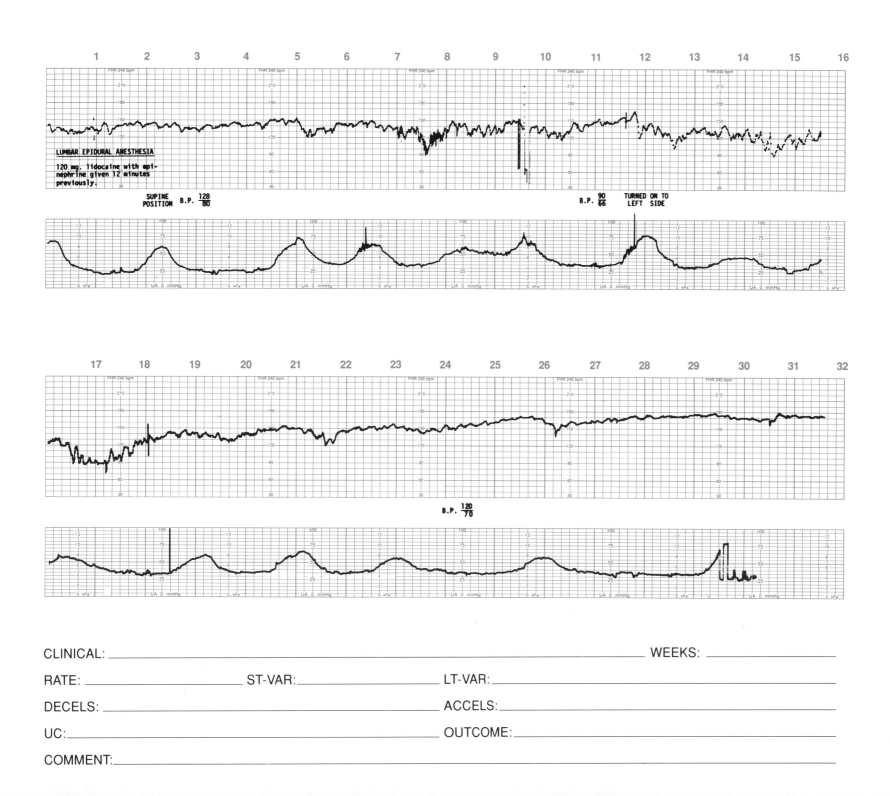

LUMBAR EPIDURAL ANESTHESIA

120 mg. lidocaine with epinephrine given 12 minutes previously.

SUPINE POSITION B.P. 128/80

B.P. 90/66   TURNED ON TO LEFT SIDE

B.P. 120/70

CLINICAL: _____ WEEKS: _____

RATE: _____ ST-VAR: _____ LT-VAR: _____

DECELS: _____ ACCELS: _____

UC: _____ OUTCOME: _____

COMMENT: _____

TRACING: 38

CLINICAL: Suspect IUGR.

WEEKS: 36

RATE: 170

STV: A: Decreased. B: Decreased.

LTV: A: Decreased. B: Decreased.

DECELERATIONS: A: Late. B: Absent.

ACCELERATIONS: A: Absent. B: Sporadic.

UC: Both: Regular—oxytocin effect.

NST: A: Nonreactive. B: Nonreactive.

CST: A: Positive. B: Negative.

OUTCOME: Growth-retarded infant; normal Apgar scores.

COMMENT: The *upper panel* was obtained during a CST with an oxytocin infusion rate of 10 mU/min. Each contraction elicits a recurrent, uniform, symmetric, late deceleration—a positive CST. In addition, the baseline rate is elevated (about 170 bpm) and both variability and accelerations are absent. Despite the considerable artifact in the first 3 minutes, recovery from the late deceleration is clearly discernible. It is inappropriate to argue that this artifact precludes determining whether a deceleration is present or not.

The *lower panel* was obtained with a direct electrode 3 hours later during the induction of labor with oxytocin running at 3 mU/min. Decelerations are absent and there is abundant short-term variability but little long-term variability. The designation "good variability" refers to the presence of adequate short-term variability. The simultaneous absence of long-term variability is of little consequence. A minimal deceleration, probably variable, appears at 22M and is not repeated. Although a sporadic acceleration appears at 29M, this panel would be classified as a nonreactive NST/negative CST.

In both panels, the contractions reflect the effect of oxytocin, i.e., they tend to be regular with similar amplitudes, durations, and intervals. This infant was delivered vaginally several hours later. Though manifestly growth-retarded and meconium-stained, the Apgar scores were satisfactory and the neonatal course and follow-up were normal.

How should we classify this test result? Because the fetus tolerated labor without late decelerations, the first temptation is to refer to the positive CST as "false-positive." But this "false-positive" test result certainly detected an abnormality, prompted intervention, and likely contributed to the salutary outcome. The absence of late decelerations in the second panel may represent: (1) a reduced level of stress (oxytocin, contractions, anxiety, aortocaval compression, etc.) with improvement in the condition of the fetus; (2) an effect of ruptured membranes; (3) misinterpretation of the tracing. There is no obvious explanation in this case.

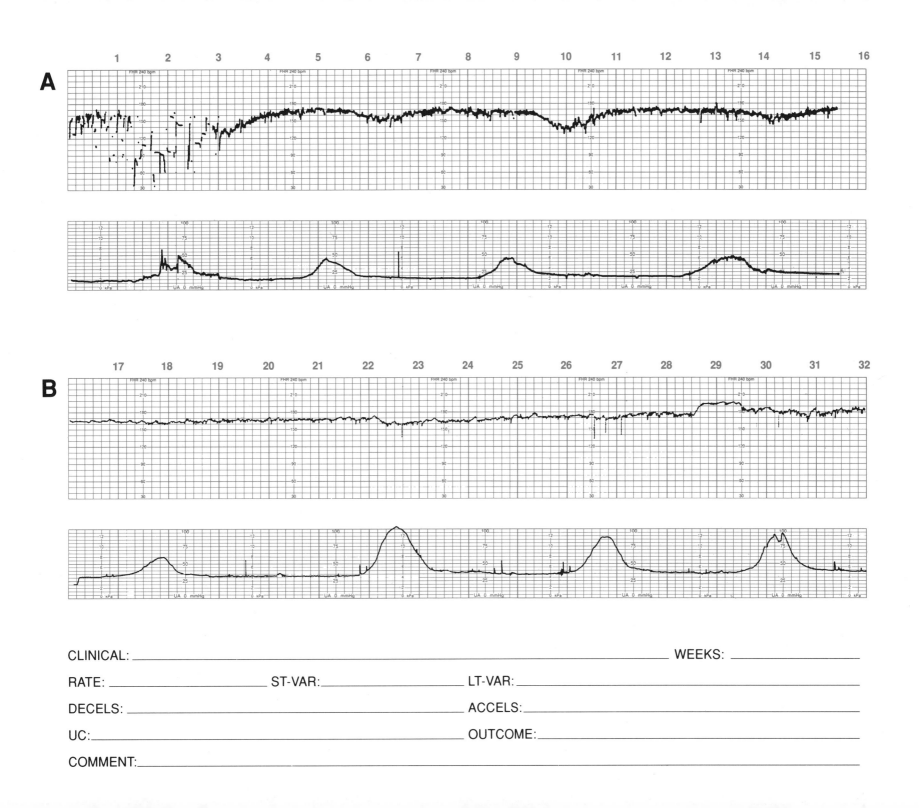

CLINICAL: _____ WEEKS: _____

RATE: _____ ST-VAR: _____ LT-VAR: _____

DECELS: _____ ACCELS: _____

UC: _____ OUTCOME: _____

COMMENT: _____

TRACING: 39

CLINICAL: Uterus didelphys; size less than dates.

WEEKS: 37

RATE: 140

STV: Absent.

LTV: Absent.

DECELERATIONS: Late.

ACCELERATIONS: Absent.

UC: Frequent, coupling.

NST: Nonreactive.

CST: Positive.

OUTCOME: Neonatal death.

COMMENT: This tracing reveals an ominous combination of absent accelerations, decreased variability (despite the considerable artifact), and recurrent late decelerations. When the late decelerations drop below 70 or 60 bpm they induce the monitor to double-count the heart rate. This produces the totally improbable appearance at 21M and 28M. Double counting develops between 50 and 100 bpm, depending on the machine and to some extent on the rhythmic pattern of the fetal heart at low rates. Contractions are somewhat irregular and tend to couple. There is considerable artifact and maternal movement on the UC tracing which produces no obvious effect on the fetal rate. At delivery, this meconium-stained infant had Apgar scores of 1 and 0 and died in the neonatal period.

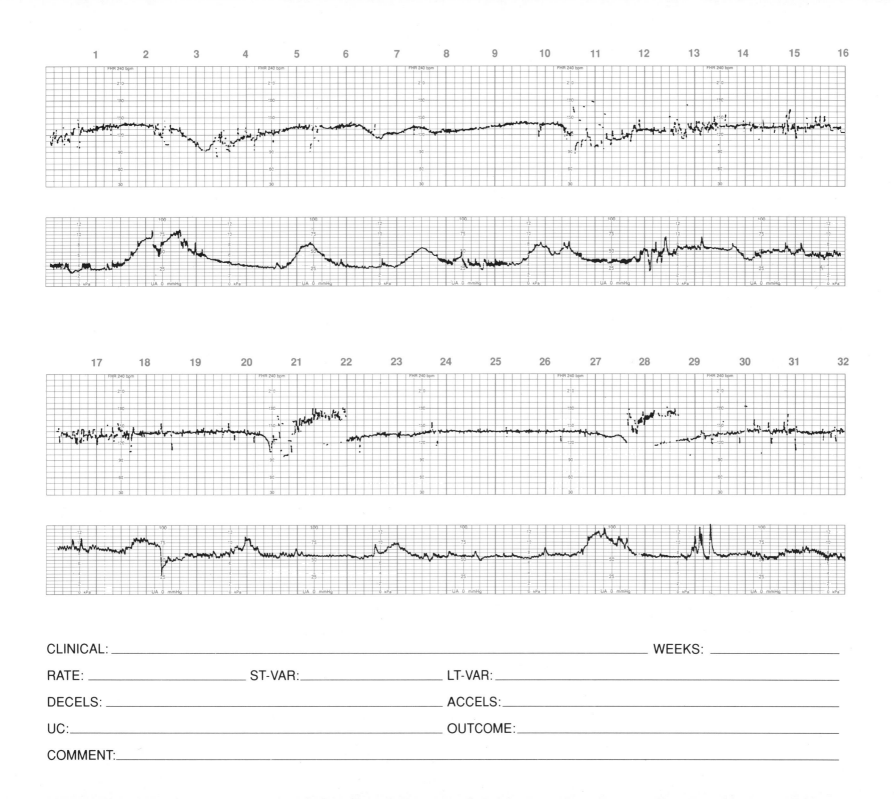

CLINICAL: _____ WEEKS: _____

RATE: _____ ST-VAR: _____ LT-VAR: _____

DECELS: _____ ACCELS: _____

UC: _____ OUTCOME: _____

COMMENT: _____

TRACING: 40

CLINICAL: Postdate pregnancy.

WEEKS: 41

RATE: 130

STV: Absent.

LTV: Absent.

DECELERATIONS: Late.

ACCELERATIONS: Absent.

UC: Occasional.

NST: Nonreactive.

CST: Positive.

OUTCOME: Maternal-fetal transfusion; neonatal death.

COMMENT: This patient was tested at 41 weeks' gestation. The tracing reveals an absence of reactivity, a ruler-flat baseline and recurrent late decelerations associated with infrequent spontaneous contractions. Despite the infrequency of contractions it seems quite inappropriate to classify this test result as other than nonreactive/positive. Using oxytocin or breast stimulation to induce more contractions seems quite inappropriate.

Immediate cesarean section revealed a pale infant with a hemoglobin of 3 g/dL, who would die in the neonatal period. The cause of this clinically silent fetal problem was fetal-maternal transfusion.

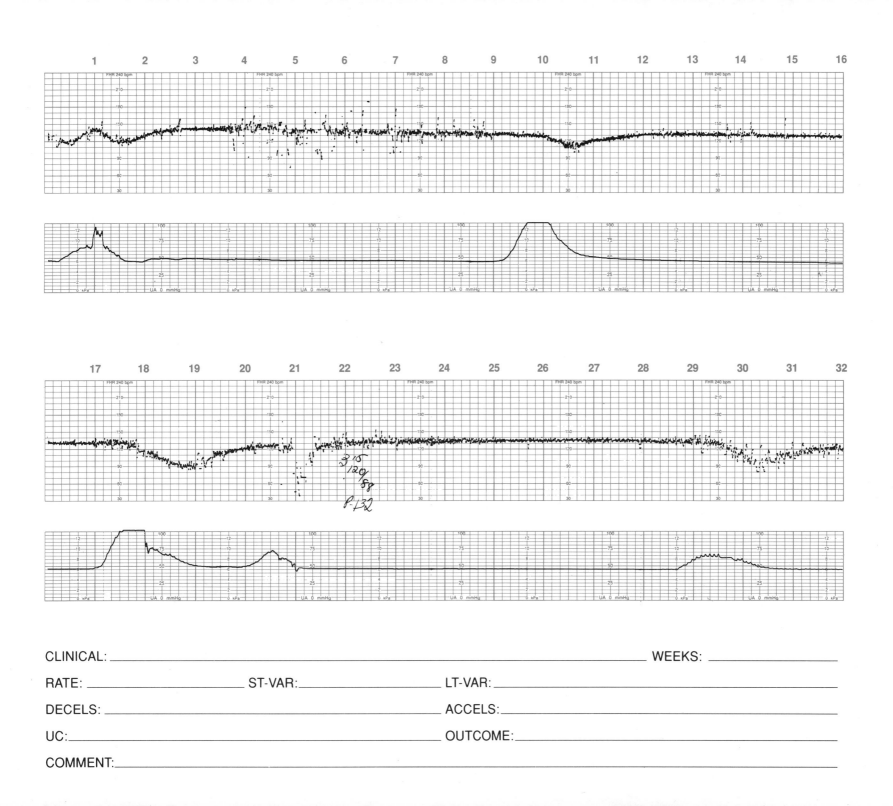

CLINICAL: _____ WEEKS: _____

RATE: _____ ST-VAR:_____ LT-VAR:_____

DECELS: _____ ACCELS:_____

UC:_____ OUTCOME:_____

COMMENT:_____

TRACING: 41

CLINICAL: Absent fetal movement.

WEEKS: 38

RATE: 150 and unstable.

STV: Absent.

LTV: Absent.

DECELERATIONS: Prolonged, ominous.

ACCELERATIONS: Absent.

UC: Oxytocin.

NST: Nonreactive.

CST: Functionally positive.

OUTCOME: Neonatal death.

COMMENT: This tracing provides additional pitfalls in the analysis of external heart rate tracings. Despite the considerable artifact due to the external ultrasound tracing, variability is absent; i.e., all the apparent variability represents artifact. The evaluation of variability with external devices (especially older monitors) is fraught with difficulty. Certain clues, however, provide insight into the true state of variability. Normal variability tends to show both long- and short-term oscillations. Long-term changes tend to be predictable while short-term variability appears almost random. The first clue, therefore, to the absent variability is the ab-

sence of accelerations. Second, the variations are not random. They derive from a consistent rate, are abrupt, and almost all the changes are downward—few are upward. In addition, we find broad, recurrent decelerations. These features should strongly suggest the absence of variability.

The baseline rate is unstable, especially in the *lower panel*. These decelerations recover only slowly, usually occupying the entire interval between contractions. Smaller contractions tend to have no added impact. This constellation of findings anticipates significant neonatal compromise. The patient delivered a hopelessly compromised infant shortly after this tracing. Only in the terminal phase of fetal deterioration do decelerations become prolonged.

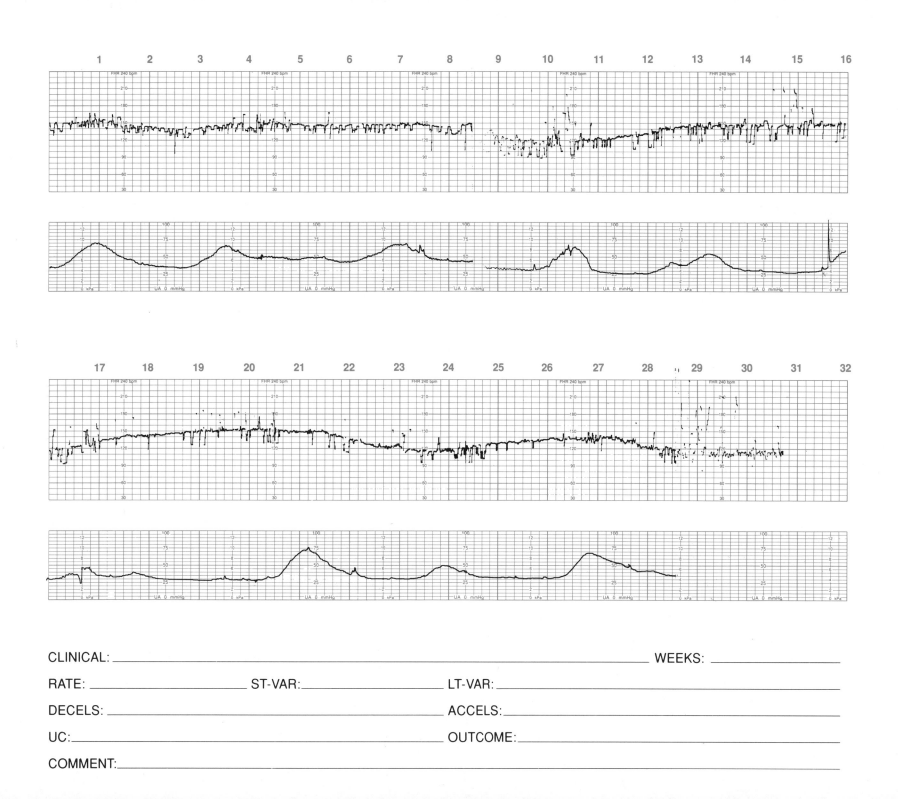

CLINICAL: _____ WEEKS: _____

RATE: _____ ST-VAR: _____ LT-VAR: _____

DECELS: _____ ACCELS: _____

UC: _____ OUTCOME: _____

COMMENT: _____

TRACING: 42

CLINICAL: Postdate pregnancy

WEEKS: 41+

BASELINE RATE: 140

STV: Upper: Average. Lower: Decreased.

LTV: Upper: Increased. Lower: Absent.

DECELERATIONS: Upper: None. Lower: Late.

ACCELERATIONS: Upper: Abundant. Lower: None.

UC: Upper: None (fetal movement). Lower: q3–4min.

OUTCOME: Cesarean section; Apgar scores 1/4; neurologic injury.

COMMENT: The *upper panel* reveals a reactive NST with ample fetal movement at 41½ weeks. Abundant accelerations accompany fetal movements and there is a clear change in behavioral state at 9M. These features strongly suggest that there is no fetal indication for intervention at this time. The clinicians were appropriately reassured and ordered repeat testing in 4 days. NST testing (with or without CST testing) is today considered inadequate for the evaluation of the postdate pregnancy. Here evaluation must also consider amniotic fluid volume.

The *lower panel* reflects an NST with spontaneous contractions (a CST) 5 days later. The pattern could not be more different. Baseline variability is decreased and accelerations are absent. In addition, each spontaneous contraction produces a late deceleration proportional in amplitude to the contraction. The deceleration associated with the third contraction is interrupted by artifact. This represents a nonreactive NST and positive CST and warrants immediate delivery. Some believe that this pattern, especially in the postdate pregnancy, requires immediate delivery by cesarean section. Others agree on the need for intervention but believe that labor may be induced with careful surveillance, because these patterns may occasionally revert to more normal tracings and the decelerations disappear. The disagreement is moot as most fetuses with this pattern during antepartum testing will simply show an identical or worse pattern in labor necessitating prompt cesarean section. In this case, however, no intervention was undertaken—with disastrous results. See tracing 43.

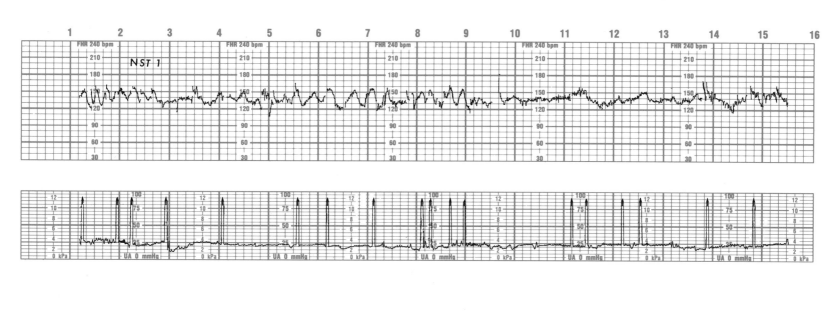

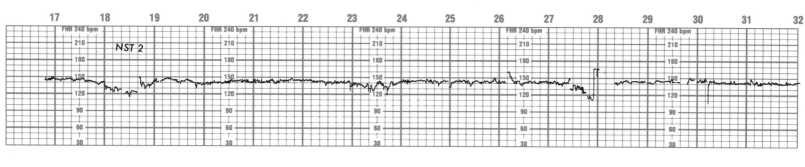

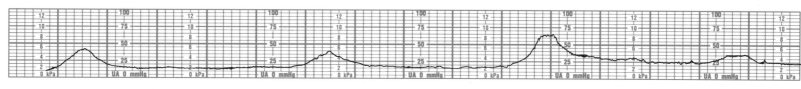

CLINICAL: _____ WEEKS: _____

RATE: _____ ST-VAR: _____ LT-VAR: _____

DECELS: _____ ACCELS: _____

UC: _____ OUTCOME: _____

COMMENT: _____

TRACING: 43

CLINICAL: PIH, thick meconium, labor.

WEEKS: 42+

BASELINE RATE: 140

STV: Absent.

LTV: Average (sinsusoidal).

DECELERATIONS: Variable with overshoot; sinusoidal.

ACCELERATIONS: None.

UC: Early labor.

OUTCOME: Cesarean section; Apgar scores 1/4; macrosomia; neurologic injury.

COMMENT: This tracing, obtained 1 day after the *lower panel* of tracing 42, reveals absent variability, intermittent undulations in the baseline (sinusoidal pattern), mild variable decelerations with overshoot, and no obvious decelerations with minimal contractions. These features represent the chronic pattern and strongly suggest neurologic injury.

The *lower tracing,* obtained later in labor with a direct electrode, reveals a similar pattern. Note that decelerations are absent except for the deceleration at 26M. The reader should resist the temptation to call this change a "late deceleration," subtle or otherwise, as the pattern does not repeat. Reasonably, despite the likely diagnosis of neurologic injury there is no ongoing asphyxia. Whether this tracing now requires cesarean delivery involves a complex set of medical, ethical, and legal considerations, answers to which are only presently evolving.

Tracings 42 and 43 reasonably reveal the progression from reactive NST with normal fetal behavior to a nonreactive NST/positive CST with decreased variability and late decelerations (asphyxia) and finally to a chronic pattern revealing a neurologically injured, but now nonasphyxiated fetus. What can be said about the recoverability of the abnormal behavior and asphyxia in the *lower panel* in tracing 42? At the present time, no conclusions are possible; the tracing that contains ongoing asphyxia cannot simultaneously be interpreted for its ultimate neurologic handicap. Once the asphyxia has ameliorated, the pattern may be used to infer adverse neurologic outcome. In a recent study, we have shown that the majority of patients with a chronic pattern during labor have reactive NSTs within 1 week of labor.

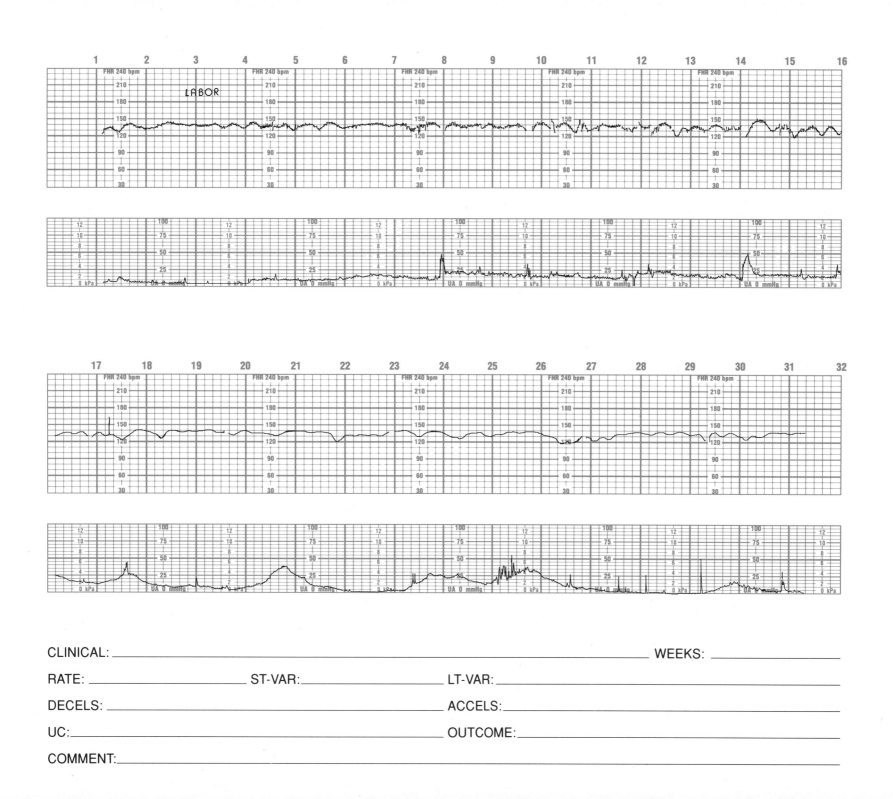

LABOR

CLINICAL: _____ WEEKS: _____

RATE: _____ ST-VAR: _____ LT-VAR: _____

DECELS: _____ ACCELS: _____

UC: _____ OUTCOME: _____

COMMENT: _____

TRACING: 44

CLINICAL: Both: Uterine hypertonus.

WEEKS: 40

BASELINE RATE: A: 150   B: 150

STV: A: Average. B: Decreased.

LTV: A: Exaggerated. B: Decreased.

DECELERATIONS: A: Variable. B: Variable, prolonged.

ACCELERATIONS: Both: None

UC: Hypertonus.

OUTCOME: Both: Apparently normal. B: Should receive follow-up.

COMMENT: These tracings illustrate qualitative differences in the fetal heart rate pattern of prolonged decelerations. In the *upper panel* the patient is unmedicated. Contractions are frequent, variability is exaggerated (saltatory), and decelerations are absent. The fetus responds to the excessive uterine activity between 5M and 10M with an erratic but prolonged deceleration. As the contractions space out, the fetal heart rate begins to return and then surpass the previous baseline for a brief period which is proportional to the duration of the fetal hypoxemia. Often the fetus exhibits one or more late decelerations during the recovery (at 12M). The nadir of the deceleration never goes below 90 bpm and the fetus retains considerable variability during the deceleration. In the *lower panel* the mother has been medicated and the variability, less dramatic than in the *upper panel,* is nevertheless quite normal. In response to the obvious uterine tetany, the fetal heart rate plummets to about 60–70 bpm with absent variability. This represents nodal rhythm; its development is a function of the responsiveness of the fetus, the severity and rapidity of the insult, and the medication administered to the mother. As the contractions space out, the heart rate begins its recovery but is interrupted by several late decelerations. The fetus will have sustained tachycardia and decreased variability. The fetus will never recover to the previous baseline rate and variability, suggesting injury from the hypoxemic stress. In both cases, clinical management should include cessation of oxytocin, repositioning to the left side, and administration of tocolytics to effectively diminish the uterine activity and promote optimum maternal-fetal circulatory exchange.

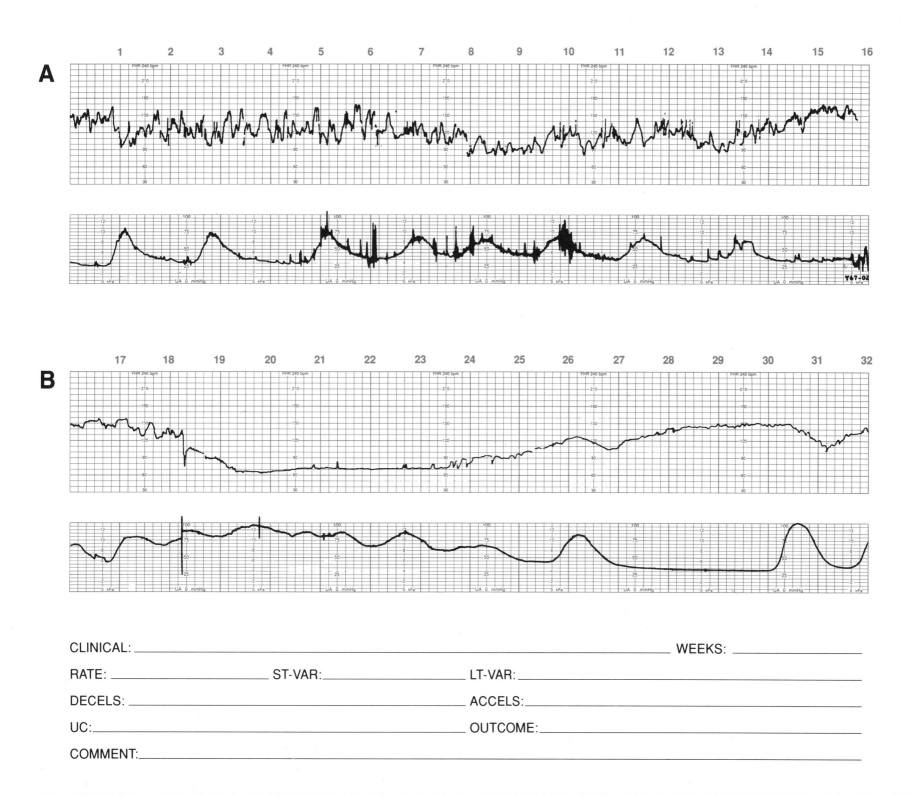

A

B

CLINICAL: _____ WEEKS: _____

RATE: _____ ST-VAR: _____ LT-VAR: _____

DECELS: _____ ACCELS: _____

UC: _____ OUTCOME: _____

COMMENT: _____

TRACING: 45

CLINICAL: Paracervical block

WEEKS: 40

BASELINE RATE: 140

STV: Decreased.

LTV: Decreased.

DECELERATIONS: Prolonged.

ACCELERATIONS: Isolated; lambda.

UC: Oxytocin; hypertonus.

OUTCOME: Apparently normal; Apgar scores, 8, 9.

COMMENT: From the outset, this tracing exhibits a markedly stable baseline heart rate with decreased variability. Paracervical block is administered at 2–4M. Beginning at 9M, small nondescript accelerations appear. At about 17M, 15 minutes after the administration of the PCB, there begins an episode of uterine hypertonus. This is an infrequent response to PCB, but is the most common response associated with PCB bradycardia. A pelvic examination during the deceleration produces some artifact and some brief accelerations in the heart rate (attempts at recovery?). The pattern recovers (after this tracing) to the previous baseline without tachycardia, indicating a lack of significant hypoxemia or damage from this particular episode. The overall pattern, however, is not reassuring.

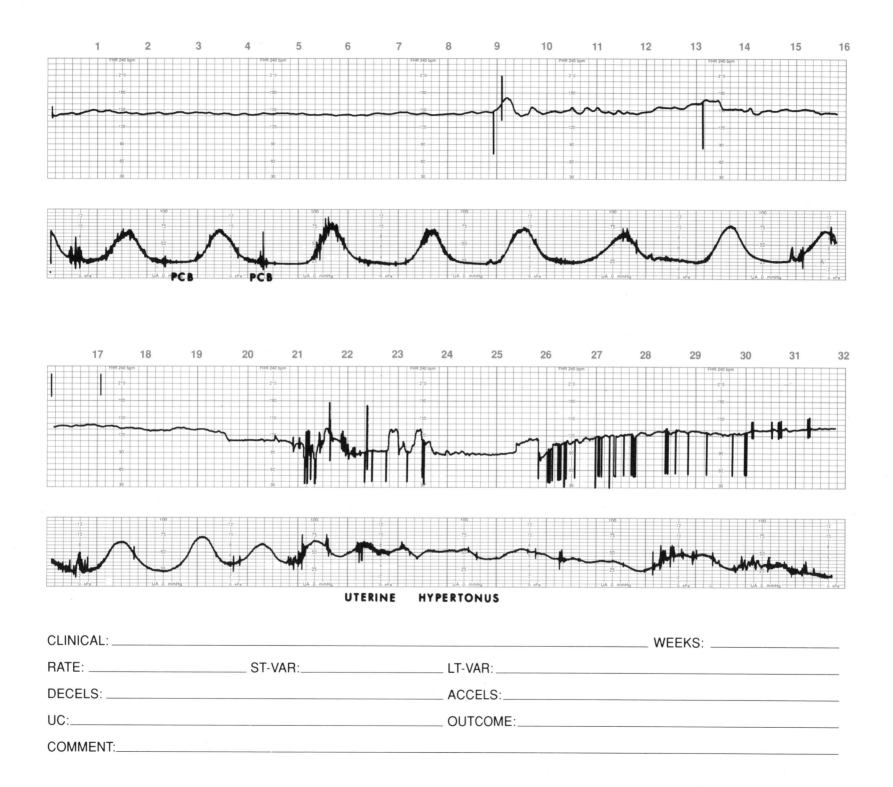

UTERINE HYPERTONUS

CLINICAL:_____ WEEKS:_____

RATE:_____ ST-VAR:_____ LT-VAR:_____

DECELS:_____ ACCELS:_____

UC:_____ OUTCOME:_____

COMMENT:_____

TRACING: 46

CLINICAL: Uneventful pregnancy

WEEKS: 40

BASELINE RATE: Upper: 130   Lower: 160

STV: Average.

LTV: Upper: Average. Lower: Increased (sinusoidal).

DECELERATIONS: Absent.

ACCELERATIONS: Sporadic.

UC: Labor.

OUTCOME: Meconium staining; neonatal sepsis; normal.

COMMENT: The *upper panel* reflects a normal reactive term fetus with a baseline of 120 bpm and numerous accelerations, epochal behavior, and absent decelerations. The UC channel reflects a "normally reactive," unmedicated mother. Because of the mother's activity and discomfort, the quality of the recording is poor and the contractions are difficult to discern. Prior to the *lower panel*, the patient received epidural anesthesia using 0.5% bupivacaine with epinephrine. The early part of this panel reflects the pharmacologic effects of both drugs. As a generaliza- tion, local anesthetics decrease variability in the fetal heart rate while epinephrine tends to elevate the rate, sometimes producing the oscillatory changes seen here. This represents no fetal compromise—just the effect of the drugs. At about 30 minutes, the patient became hypotensive necessitating the use of intravenous ephedrine (see next tracing). Note how much easier it is to see the contractions after the patient has received her medication.

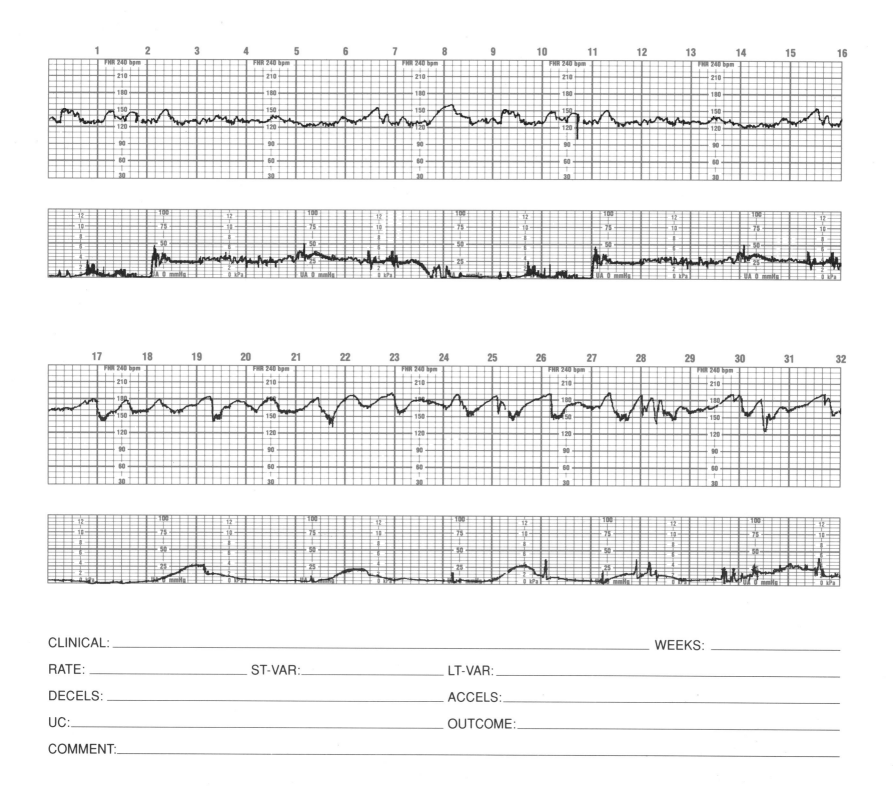

CLINICAL: _____   WEEKS: _____

RATE: _____ ST-VAR: _____   LT-VAR: _____

DECELS: _____   ACCELS: _____

UC: _____   OUTCOME: _____

COMMENT: _____

TRACING: 47

CLINICAL: Hypotension following epidural anesthesia; ephedrine.

WEEKS: 40

BASELINE RATE: 190

STV: Average.

LTV: Increased.

DECELERATIONS: Mild variable.

ACCELERATIONS: Saltatory.

UC: Irregular.

OUTCOME: Meconium staining; neonatal sepsis; normal.

COMMENT: This tracing represents a continuation of tracing 46. The *upper panel* reveals the dramatic exaggeration of the previous oscillatory pattern. The frequency and the amplitude of the baseline changes have increased dramatically—a saltatory pattern. While this pattern may appear spontaneously (see tracings 23 and 27), it is commonly seen following the administration of ephedrine (Clark RB, Brunner JA: *Anesthesiology* 53:514–517, 1980). The pattern changes somewhat after the 2 small variable decelerations at 8M and 9M. The baseline is higher, and the amplitude and frequency of the oscillations lower.

The *lower panel* shows the resolution of the saltatory pattern although the tachycardia persists for some time. Barring any adverse events or anesthetic effect, this tracing may be expected to resume its previous reassuring pattern when the effects of the ephedrine have worn off and the fetus has had adequate recovery time. The effects of the medication on both the fetal heart rate and pattern will last for about 1 hour. Ephedrine, like epinephrine, also diminishes uterine activity.

This mother will develop fever and chorioamnionitis later in labor as a result of group B streptococcal infection.

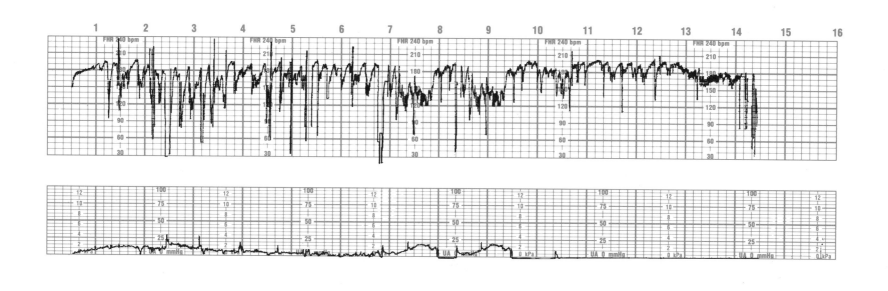

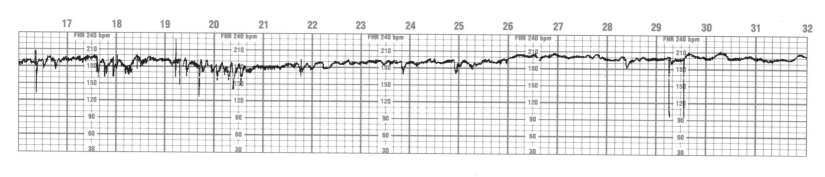

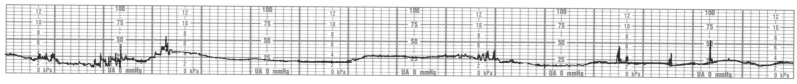

CLINICAL:_____ WEEKS:_____

RATE:_____ ST-VAR:_____ LT-VAR:_____

DECELS:_____ ACCELS:_____

UC:_____ OUTCOME:_____

COMMENT:_____

TRACING: 48

CLINICAL: Uneventful pregnancy, OP position.

WEEKS: 37

BASELINE RATE: 150

STV: Average.

LTV: Average.

DECELERATIONS: Variable, prolonged.

ACCELERATIONS: Isolated; shoulders.

UC: Oxytocin, hypertonus

OUTCOME: Midforceps delivery; Apgar scores 7/8; neurologic injury.

COMMENT: This tracing, running at a paper speed of 1 cm/min, reveals a reassuring fetal pattern in response to oxytocin stimulation. Until 21M the baseline rate is quite stable and the variability is average. Either accelerations or brief variable decelerations with shoulders accompany contractions. The contractions tend to be regularly spaced and of similar amplitude—an effect of oxytocin. Beginning at 21M the fetus responds to the exaggerated uterine activity with a prolonged deceleration, evolving through a series of late decelerations into an episode of compensatory tachycardia. By the end of the panel, the heart rate is returning to its previous baseline and periodic accelerations are present. This represents a period of fetal hypoxemia related to uterine hypertonus from which the fetus appears to recover. The severity of the episode is estimated by the duration of the compensatory tachycardia. Reasonably, by the end of the panel, the fetus has recovered completely from the episode. This tracing continues in tracing 49.

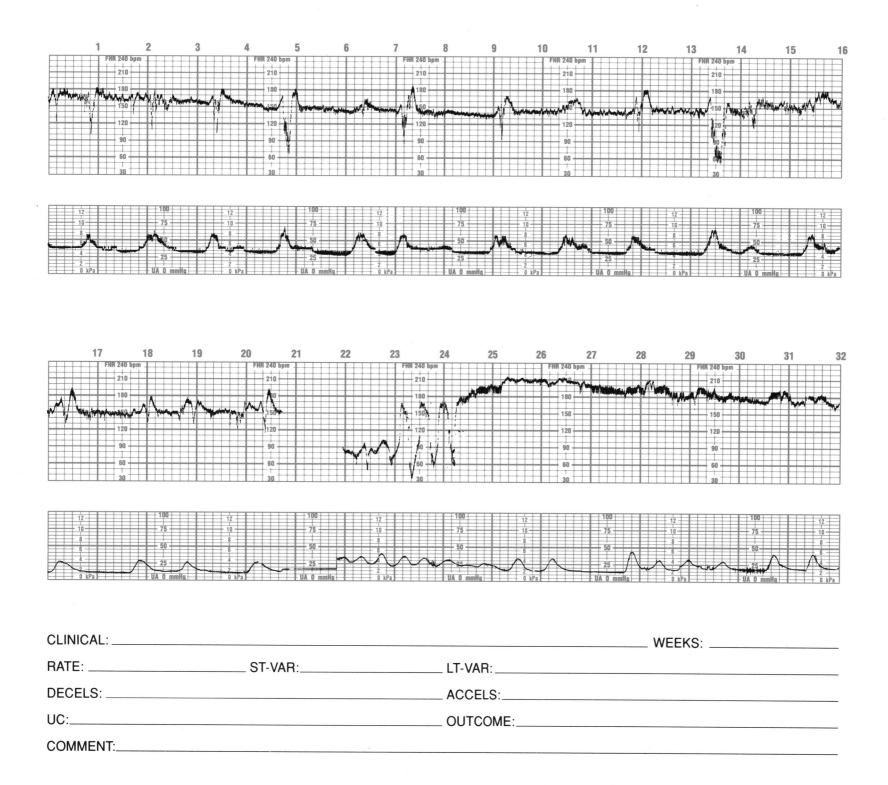

CLINICAL: _____ WEEKS: _____

RATE: _____ ST-VAR: _____ LT-VAR: _____

DECELS: _____ ACCELS: _____

UC: _____ OUTCOME: _____

COMMENT: _____

TRACING: 49

CLINICAL: OP labor; meperidine (Demerol).

WEEKS: 37

BASELINE RATE: Upper: 160   Lower: 180

STV: Decreased.

LTV: Decreased.

DECELERATIONS: Variable, prolonged.

ACCELERATIONS: Isolated.

UC: Oxytocin, bearing down.

OUTCOME: Midforceps delivery; Apgar scores 7/8; neurologic injury.

COMMENT: This tracing, continued from tracing 48 (still at 1 cm/min paper speed), begins with continuing frequent uterine contractions with occasional runs of polysystole. The fetus responds to most contractions with accelerations; the variability is somewhat diminished. At 11M, in association with an attempt to manually dilate the cervix, the fetus responds with a series of prolonged variable decelerations. In response to these decelerations, the baseline rate increases and variability apparently decreases (see *lower panel*). In contrast to the events in tracing 48 where the prolonged deceleration is followed by a transient tachycardia, here the baseline rate remains elevated and fetal reactivity never returns. Almost 90 minutes later (at 26M), in association with frequent contractions and bearing-down efforts, the fetus develops a series of variable decelerations that on recovery (at 30M) seem to raise the baseline even higher. Smaller decel-erations persist until the end of the tracing. The infant was somewhat depressed at birth, had convulsions soon after delivery, and showed residual neurologic deficit.

In aggregate, the tracings suggest a previously normal fetus subjected to several hypoxemic episodes. The fetus recovers completely (from acid-base and neurologic perspectives) from the first episode (tracing 48) but never recovers from the second episode, when it is later subject to a third episode. Reasonably then, the subsequent neurologic handicap relates to these events in labor.

The OP position is implicated in abnormal labor curves and adverse outcome more often than OA. This position is often associated with variable decelerations due to tremendous head compression during the second stage. Whether OP position is the cause, the result, or simply a correlative finding of neurologic injury, it is well to treat all laboring women with OP position with the utmost caution and consideration of the potential for difficult vaginal delivery.

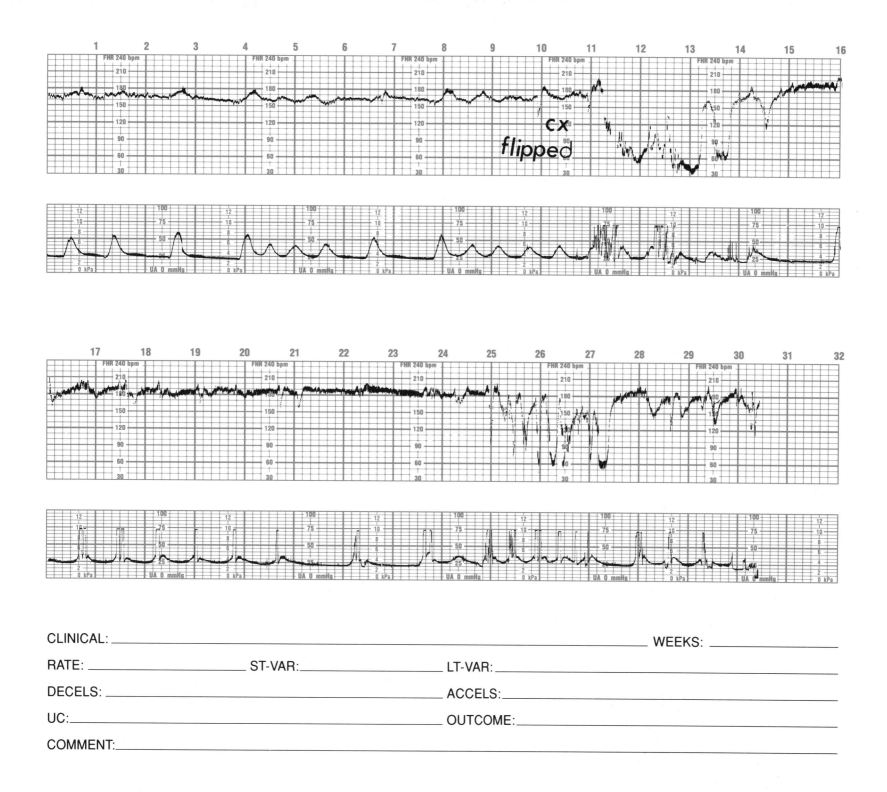

cx
flipped

CLINICAL: _____ WEEKS: _____

RATE: _____ ST-VAR: _____ LT-VAR: _____

DECELS: _____ ACCELS: _____

UC: _____ OUTCOME: _____

COMMENT: _____

TRACING: 50

CLINICAL: OP labor.

WEEKS: 39

BASELINE RATE: 150

STV: Average.

LTV: Average.

DECELERATIONS: Variable.

ACCELERATIONS: Shoulders.

UC: Oxytocin, bearing down.

OUTCOME: Meconium aspiration syndrome.

COMMENT: This and the subsequent tracing illustrate the deterioration of variable decelerations in the second stage of labor with the fetus in the OP position. In this tracing, we find frequent uterine contractions with occasional coupling arousing suspicion of placental abruption. Repetitive variable decelerations with shoulders accompany each contraction. The amplitude and duration of the decelerations vary considerably, but the baseline remains stable and variability persists. With the onset of the second stage and maternal expulsive efforts (17M), the decelerations increase in amplitude and duration. Note that the amplitude of the deceleration results mostly from the rise in the baseline rather than a lower nadir. For the most part, the baseline variability remains intact. While the progressive rise in the baseline rate suggests a deterioration in fetal "reserve," the maintenance of variability suggests that the fetus is both able to compensate and remain neurologically intact. It does seem unnecessary, however, to challenge the fetus in this way. In the face of this high frequency of uterine contractions and the rising fetal baseline, it seems reasonable to at least periodically restrain the mother from pushing and allow the fetus ample time to recover.

This newborn suffered from meconium aspiration syndrome (MAS) although it ultimately did well. While the proper aspiration of the fetus at the time of delivery is thought to prevent MAS, some MAS has its genesis before labor and delivery and cannot be prevented by tracheal toilet at the time of delivery. Although no definitive connection between the events of labor, FHR patterns, and MAS has been established, variable decelerations may be associated with fetal gasping.

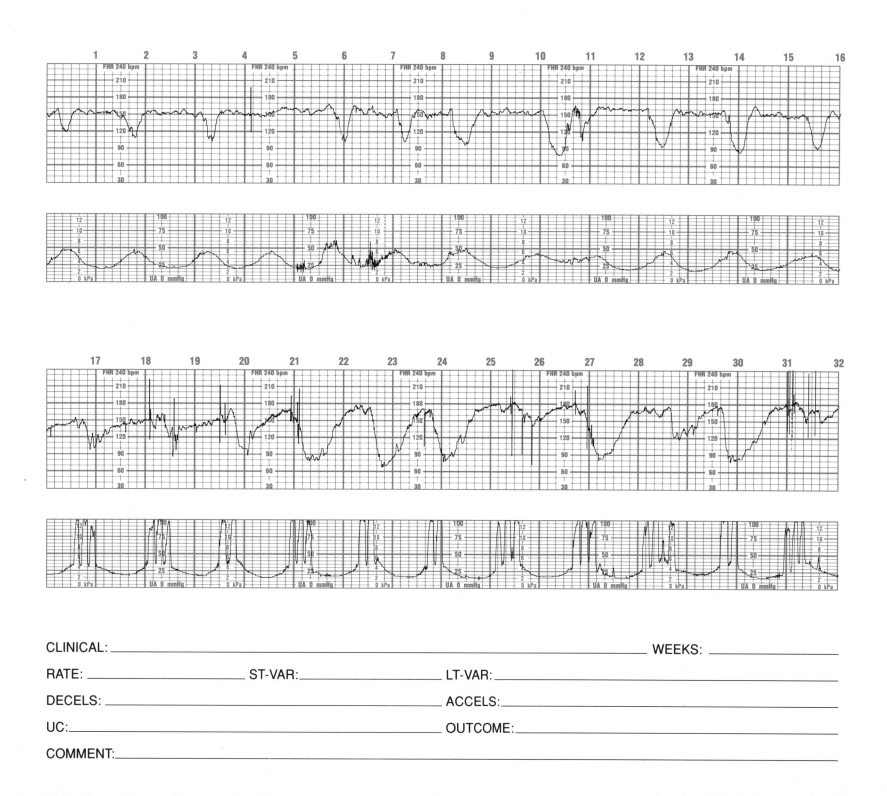

CLINICAL: _____ WEEKS: _____

RATE: _____ ST-VAR: _____ LT-VAR: _____

DECELS: _____ ACCELS: _____

UC: _____ OUTCOME: _____

COMMENT: _____

TRACING: 51

CLINICAL: Uneventful pregnancy; OP position during labor.

WEEKS: 36

BASELINE RATE: Upper: 160   Lower: 180

STV: Decreased.

LTV: Decreased.

DECELERATIONS: Variable.

ACCELERATIONS: None.

UC: Frequent UC; oxytocin effect; second stage.

OUTCOME: Apgar scores 7/9/10.

COMMENT: The tracing illustrates the progressive deterioration of the fetal tracing during the second stage of labor. The *upper panel* reveals a modestly elevated baseline rate with minimal variability. The frequent contractions elicit no decelerations. At the onset of pushing, deep variable decelerations appear with each contraction and the pattern rapidly deteriorates. The baseline rate and the amplitude of the decelerations increase. In addition, the decelerations seem to become smoother and more rounded at the bottom. By 27M the variability is flat and there is no recovery between decelerations. At this point, if not before, pushing must cease to allow the fetus to recover. Whether the source of these decelerations be cord compression, head compression, or hypoxia, none are ameliorated by pushing. At the end of this panel the patient was taken to the delivery room with the intention of expediting delivery with forceps. In the delivery room, the patient ceased pushing temporarily and the pattern recovered. The infant ultimately was delivered spontaneously, with normal Apgar scores and a cord pH of 7.23.

Head compression, not cord compression, seems the most obvious explanation of these decelerations, which begin with the onset of pushing and are relieved by cessation of pushing. Thus obvious deterioration of the tracing in this case nothwithstanding, such changes cannot be used to infer fetal injury.

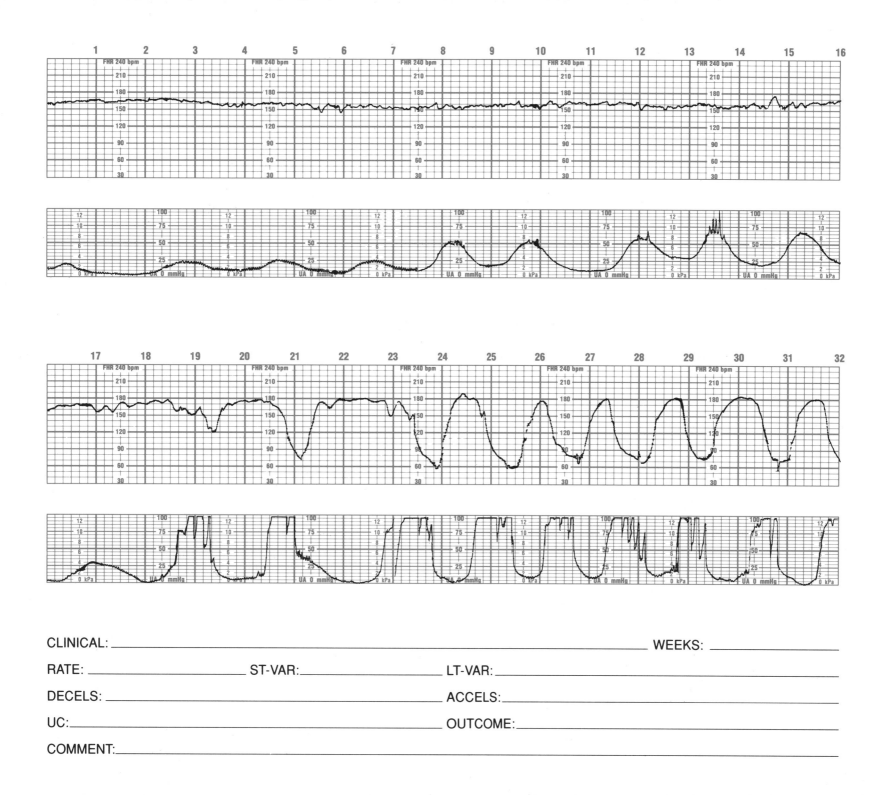

CLINICAL: _____ WEEKS: _____

RATE: _____ ST-VAR: _____ LT-VAR: _____

DECELS: _____ ACCELS: _____

UC: _____ OUTCOME: _____

COMMENT: _____

TRACING: 52

CLINICAL: Maternal chronic renal disease; prophylactic antibiotics.

WEEKS: 36

BASELINE RATE: 170–180

STV: Decreased.

LTV: Decreased.

DECELERATIONS: Variable.

ACCELERATIONS: None.

UC: Bearing down in the second stage.

OUTCOME: Spontaneous vaginal delivery; Apgar scores 7/9.

COMMENT: This tracing illustrates progressive deterioration of the FHR tracing during the second stage of labor in a fetus in OP position. The tracing begins with a somewhat elevated baseline with diminished variability but no decelerations. Uterine contractions are quite frequent (about 10 in 16 minutes—polysystole). In response to the maternal bearing-down effort and the frequent contractions, variable decelerations appear and become larger, and the tracing progressively deteriorates. By 25M, the baseline has risen, variability has disappeared, and there is virtually no recovery period between decelerations. The deterioration in this pattern requires prompt attention in the form of cessation of pushing along with oxygen and elimination of oxytocin infusion. This infant was delivered shortly after the end of the tracing, with normal Apgar scores.

OP positions are associated with longer labors, greater molding of the fetal head, and greater likelihood of variable decelerations in the second stage. They are also associated with an increased risk of perinatal mortality and morbidity. This increased risk may derive from several sources. The longer labors and the greater mechanical forces brought to bear on these fetuses may induce injury. The potentially traumatic effects of forceps rotation may also account for some of the increased risk associated with the OP position. Finally, preliminary evidence suggests that previously injured fetuses may show a predilection for the OP position during labor.

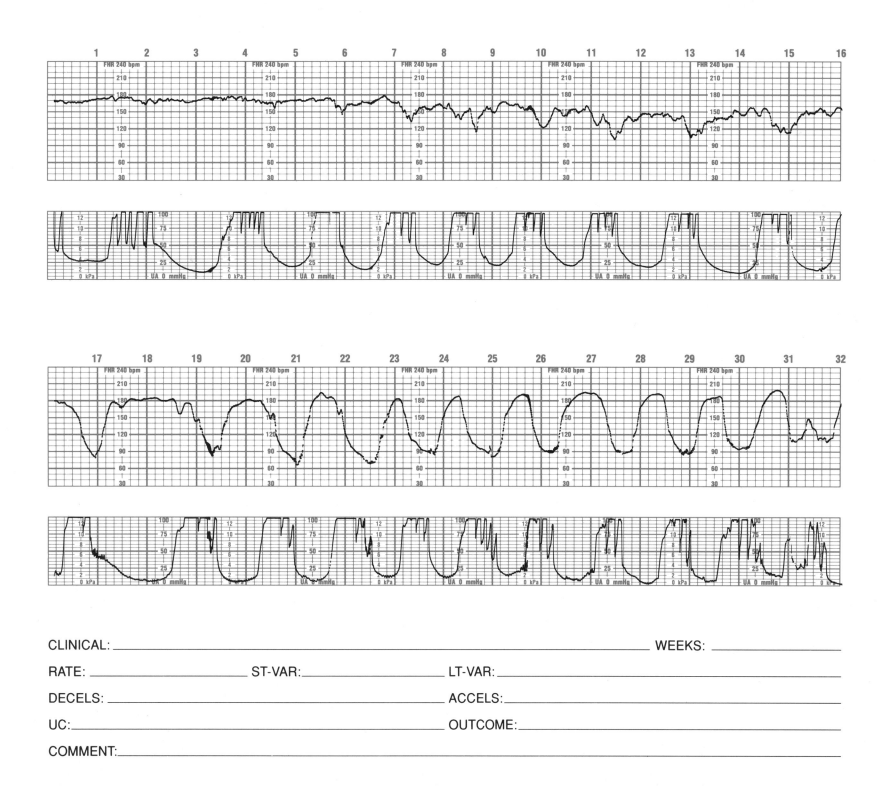

CLINICAL: _____ WEEKS: _____

RATE: _____ ST-VAR: _____ LT-VAR: _____

DECELS: _____ ACCELS: _____

UC: _____ OUTCOME: _____

COMMENT: _____

TRACING: 53

CLINICAL: Pregnancy-induced hypertension; IUGR.

WEEKS: 37

BASELINE RATE: 140

STV: Average.

LTV: Decreased.

DECELERATIONS: Variable.

ACCELERATIONS: None.

UC: Abruption.

OUTCOME: Apgar scores 5/7; neonatal seizures; neurologic injury.

COMMENT: This tracing and the subsequent one illustrate fetal deterioration to the point of neurologic injury. The *upper panel* obtained in early labor with external transducers reveals decreased variability and mild variable decelerations with frequent contractions. In the *lower panel* running at 1 cm/min, frequent contractions seem to elicit repetitive late decelerations of increasing amplitude and a rising baseline rate. The decelerations, however, are independent of the contractions. They more likely represent a neurological problem, rather than asphyxia. The maternal blood pressure at this point is quite elevated and unresponsive to hydralazine (Apresoline). In addition, she has begun to bleed vaginally. The fetal impairment may result from peripheral vasospasm or placental abruption associated with uncontrolled hypertension. Placental abruption may occasionally involve fetal bleeding. Thus, the efforts to stabilize the mother did not prevent fetal deterioration (see continuation in tracing 54).

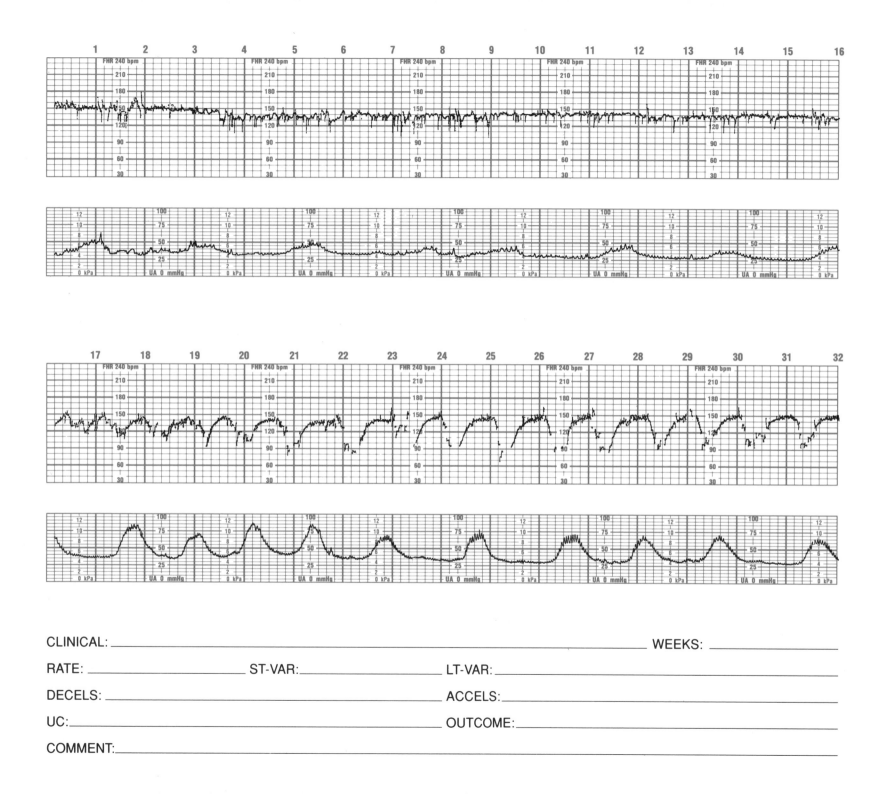

CLINICAL: _____ WEEKS: _____

RATE: _____ ST-VAR: _____ LT-VAR: _____

DECELS: _____ ACCELS: _____

UC: _____ OUTCOME: _____

COMMENT: _____

TRACING: 54

CLINICAL: PIH; hydralazine; $MgSO_4$; IUGR.

WEEKS: 37

BASELINE RATE: 160

STV: Decreased.

LTV: Absent.

DECELERATIONS: Late.

ACCELERATIONS: None.

UC: Abruption.

OUTCOME: Cesarean section; Apgar scores 5/7; neurologic injury; neonatal seizures.

COMMENT: This tracing is a continuation of tracing 53 but is recorded at 3 cm/min. Contractions have diminished but late decelerations of minimal amplitude accompany each contraction. The baseline rate is elevated and reveals absent variability, suggesting an ongoing asphyxia despite the diminution in uterine activity. In the *lower panel* the contraction frequency has decreased even further with coupling of the contractions. Decelerations continue to appear but are not so easily classifiable. The elevated baseline rate shows no variability (what is there is artifact). This entire series illustrates initially a growth-retarded but presumably salvageable fetus. The combination of placental abruption and inability to rapidly stabilize the mother resulted in the progressive asphyxiation. By the time the mother was sufficiently stabilized, the very frequent contractions had abated but the fetus was already injured. At cesarean section delivery, there was an obvious placental abruption. Nevertheless, the growth-retarded infant had reasonable Apgar scores and minimal acidosis though it did suffer neonatal seizures and subsequent cerebral palsy. In this unusual case, the uterine response to the abruption was apparently self-limited. This tracing clearly anticipates the adverse outcome for the baby.

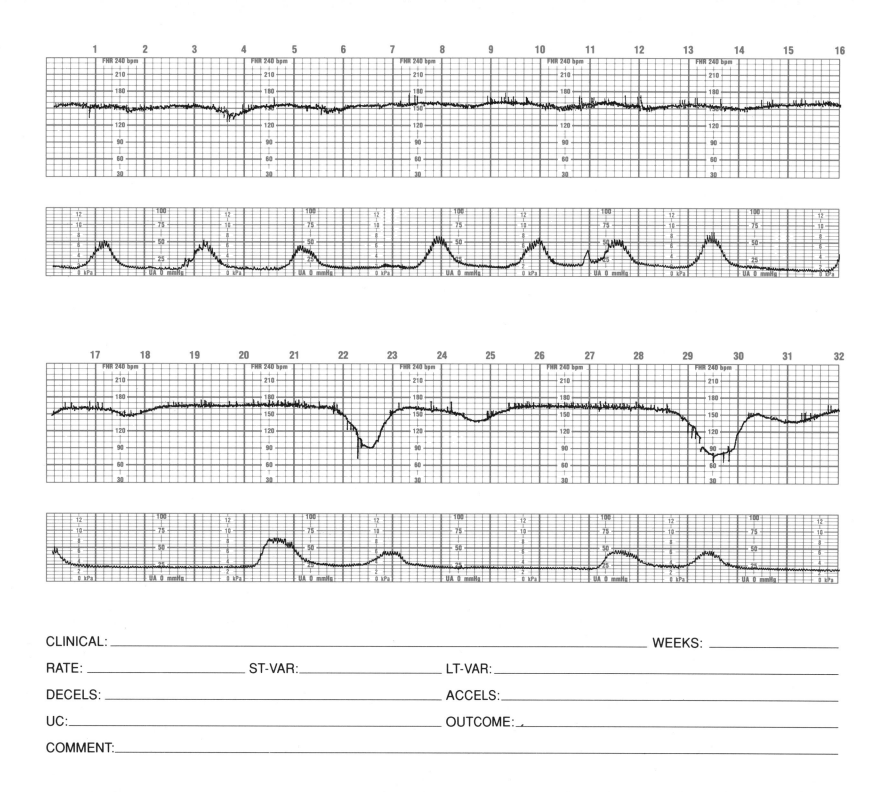

CLINICAL: _____ WEEKS: _____

RATE: _____ ST-VAR: _____ LT-VAR: _____

DECELS: _____ ACCELS: _____

UC: _____ OUTCOME: _____

COMMENT: _____

TRACING: 55

CLINICAL: Labor; meconium-stained fluid.

WEEKS: 41

BASELINE RATE: 150

STV: Decreased.

LTV: Increased.

DECELERATIONS: Variable.

ACCELERATIONS: None.

UC: Irregular; poor toco placement.

OUTCOME: Cesarean section for fetal distress;
Apgar scores 1/7; neonatal convulsions.

COMMENT: This unusual tracing reveals a stable baseline in the normal range, decreased STV, but increased LTV, especially in response to the variable decelerations in the *upper panel.* The exaggerated LTV (?sinusoidal, ?saltatory) seems to have no impact on either the baseline rate or variability and would not seem to represent an indication for delivery. In the *lower panel* there is a prolonged deceleration beginning at 18M which continues for at least 4 minutes before the heart rate begins to recover. The fetal heart rate, however, never recovers to its previous rate or pattern. The rate to which it recovers is stable and punctuated by curious excursions. Though contractions are very poorly recorded here, we may conclude that they are present but elicit no further decelerations. Understandably, the fetus was delivered by cesarean section for fetal distress. At delivery there was evidence of recent meconium. The Apgar scores were 1 and 7 after endotracheal suction of meconium; cord blood gases were normal. The infant had neonatal convulsions.

The pattern at the end of the tracing is quite similar to the "checkmark" pattern reported by Cruickshank (Cruickshank DP: An unusual fetal heart rate pattern. *Am J Obstet Gynecol* 1978; 130:101.). In that case the mother suffered cardiorespiratory arrest but was resuscitated. The fetus was later born with the "check-mark pattern," low Apgar scores, and normal cord pH values. In this case, the development of this pattern follows immediately a prolonged fetal bradycardia. Seemingly, the bradycardia may have represented either the source of the insult (hypoxia) or response to the insult.

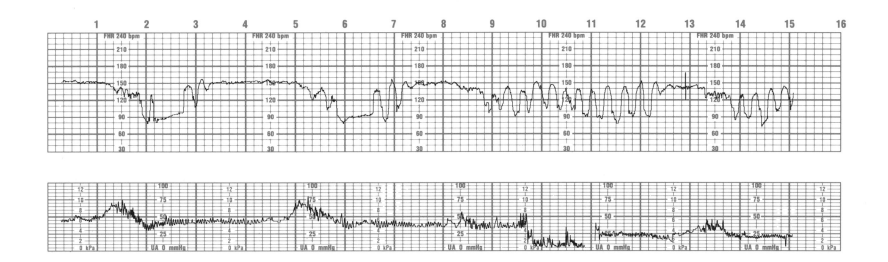

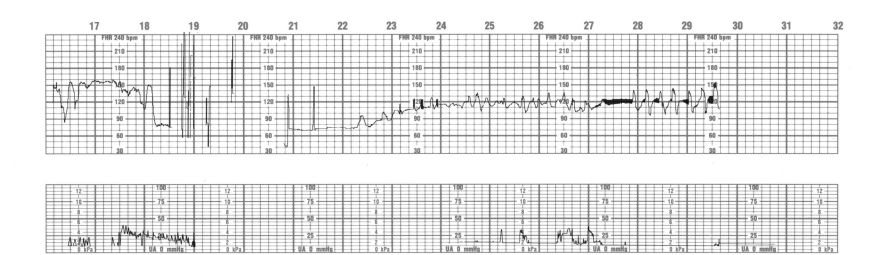

CLINICAL: _____   WEEKS: _____

RATE: _____ ST-VAR: _____ LT-VAR: _____

DECELS: _____   ACCELS: _____

UC: _____   OUTCOME: _____

COMMENT: _____

TRACING: 56

CLINICAL: Twins.

WEEKS: 36

BASELINE RATE: 145, 135

STV: Decreased.

LTV: Decreased.

DECELERATIONS: Variable in one twin, absent in the other.

ACCELERATIONS: None.

UC: None.

OUTCOME: Unknown.

COMMENT: This tracing shows a concomitantly monitored set of twins with discordant FHR patterns. One (monitored internally) has an essentially flat baseline of 145 bpm while the other, with a baseline of 135 bpm, is having spontaneous decelerations. The difference in heart rate patterns does not necessarily indicate discordant growth, but serial ultrasound examination is, of course, advised. As the differences in BPD increase, the greater the likelihood that the smaller fetus will be growth-retarded.

NSTs in twins appear to be prognostically comparable to those taken in singleton pregnancies, but in some twin cases a nonreactive NST may reflect significant distress in utero. Additionally, the presence of recurrent spontaneous decelerations with decreased variability and no accelerations, as in this case, presents strong evidence of the need for intervention. The probability of two, or even one, normal neonate resulting from this case is low.

REFERENCE

Berkowitz RL: Multiple gestations, in Gabbe SG, Niebyl JR, Simpson JL (eds): *Obstetrics, Normal and Problem Pregnancies,* New York, Churchill Livingston, 1986, pp 739–768.

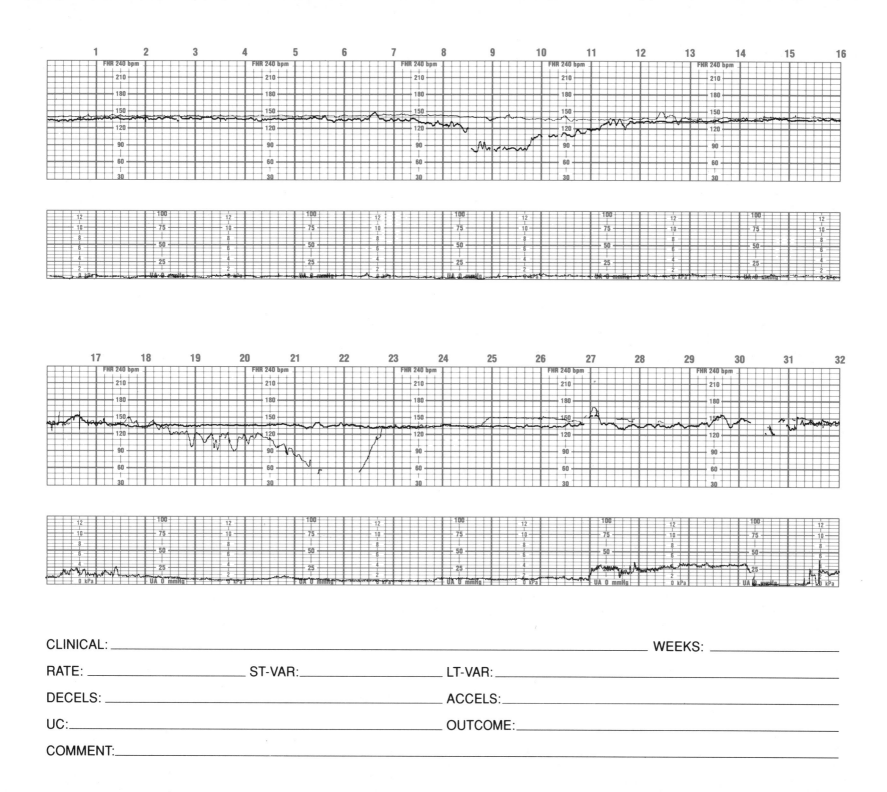

CLINICAL: _____ WEEKS: _____

RATE: _____ ST-VAR: _____ LT-VAR: _____

DECELS: _____ ACCELS: _____

UC: _____ OUTCOME: _____

COMMENT: _____

TRACING: 57

CLINICAL: Labor.

WEEKS: 41

BASELINE RATE: 120

STV: Absent.

LTV: Absent.

DECELERATIONS: Variable, late.

ACCELERATIONS: None.

UC: Oxytocin.

OUTCOME: Neurologic injury.

COMMENT: The *upper panel* reveals a ruler-flat, stable baseline with absent STV and LTV but no decelerations during labor. The differential diagnosis includes: neurologic injury, congenital anomaly involving the heart or the brain, a cardiac arrhythmia (paroxysmal supraventricular tachycardia with block), and drug effect. We can exclude asphyxia.

The *lower panel* from the same patient shows persistently absent variability along with a consistent pattern of small, paired decelerations with most of the contractions. Coinciding with the contractions we find small variable decelerations with overshoot. Late decelerations appear immediately thereafter. Toward the end of the panel, when the contractions are closer together, only the variable deceleration is found. Despite the frequent contractions and the decelerations the baseline heart rate is unchanged from the *upper panel*. This pattern, while associated with fetal injury, has not been associated with fetal asphyxia. This tracing continues in tracing 58.

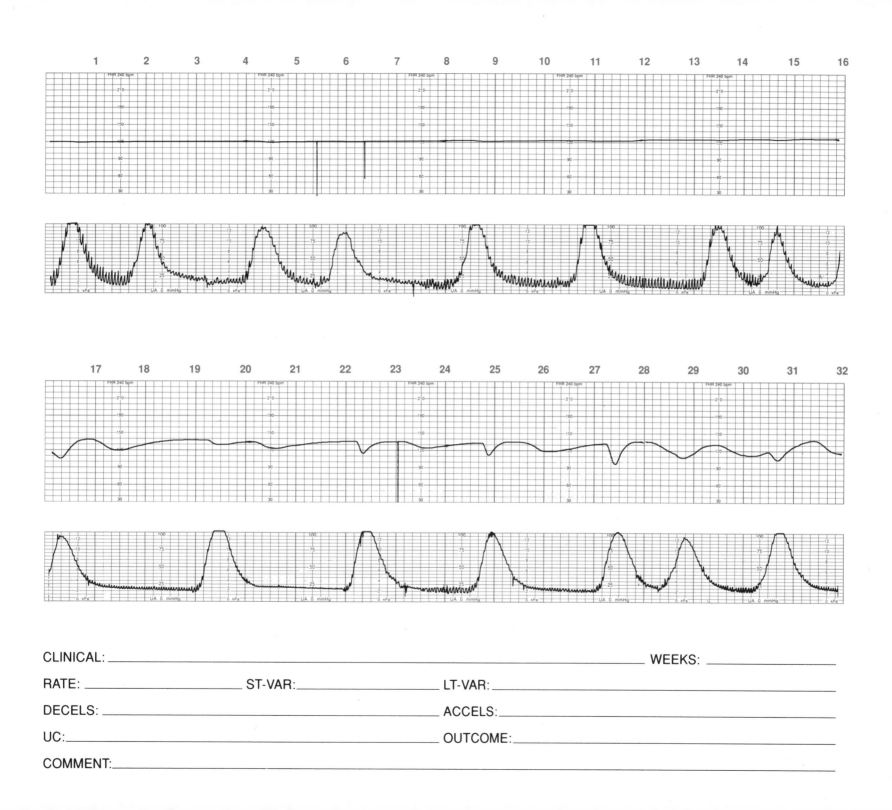

CLINICAL: _____ WEEKS: _____

RATE: _____ ST-VAR: _____ LT-VAR: _____

DECELS: _____ ACCELS: _____

UC: _____ OUTCOME: _____

COMMENT: _____

TRACING: 58

CLINICAL: Labor.

WEEKS: 41

BASELINE RATE: 130

STV: Absent.

LTV: Absent.

DECELERATIONS: Late.

ACCELERATIONS: None.

UC: Oxytocin.

OUTCOME: Oligohydramnios; meconium staining;
Apgar scores 2/6; seizures; neurologic injury.

COMMENT: This tracing follows from tracing 57 and illustrates yet other patterns in this injured fetus. In the *upper panel,* the patient has received epidural anesthesia. The small variable decelerations with overshoot have disappeared leaving only consistent, uniform late decelerations. The decelerations fulfill the major criteria for late decelerations but do not induce any change in the baseline rate. Although it is reasonable to conclude that this pattern reflects the superimposition of asphyxia onto an already injured fetus, cord gases often do not support this. In this case, by the middle of the *lower panel,* the decelerations have at least temporarily resolved as they often do spontaneously or in response to some judiciously applied oxygen and position change.

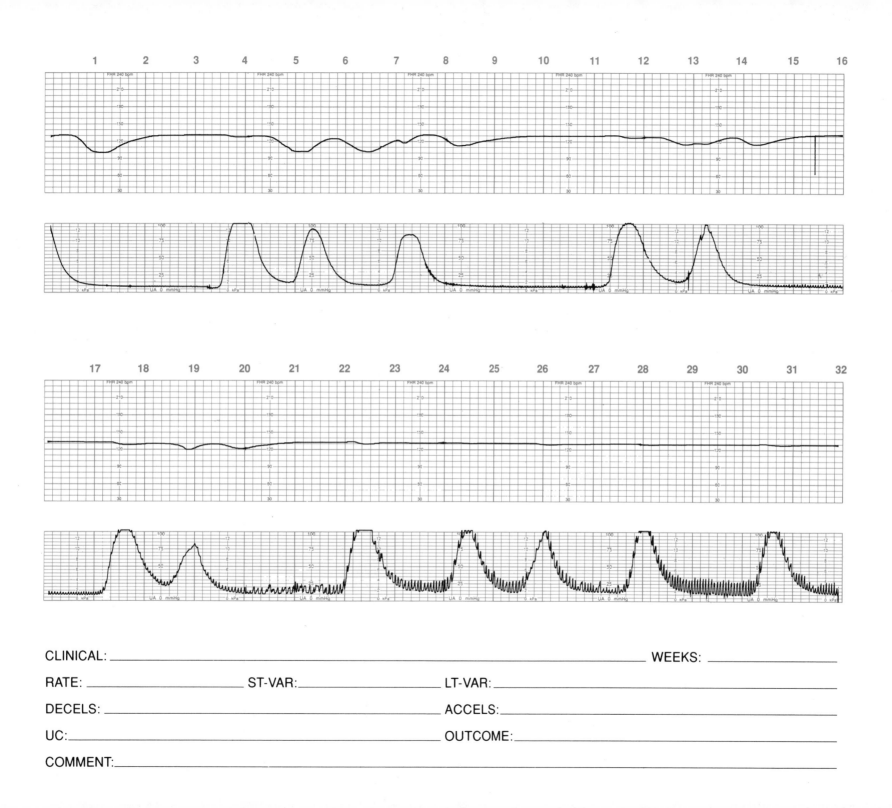

CLINICAL: _____ WEEKS: _____

RATE: _____ ST-VAR: _____ LT-VAR: _____

DECELS: _____ ACCELS: _____

UC: _____ OUTCOME: _____

COMMENT: _____

TRACING: 59

CLINICAL: Postdate pregnancy; absent fetal movement.

WEEKS: 42

RATE: 145

STV: Absent.

LTV: Absent.

DECELERATIONS: Small variable.

ACCELERATIONS: Uniform and overshoot.

UC: Coupling (tripling) with hypertonus.

NST: Nonreactive.

CST: Equivocal.

OUTCOME: Low Apgar scores (5/8); ultimate cerebral palsy.

COMMENT: This is a chronically affected, postdate fetus who, upon delivery, will show evidence of neonatal depression, meconium staining, and obvious wasting. The infant will exhibit seizures in the neonatal period and go on to develop handicapping cerebral palsy. Note the obvious absence of baseline variability and the appearance of accelerations with induced uterine contractions. The apparent decelerations at 18M, 29M, and 30M represent recovery from the accelerations (lambda patterns) and not late decelerations. Occasionally, diagnostic, small decelerations with overshoot become manifest, particularly just preceding 24M and between 27M and 28M. This most disturbing pattern, despite its unfortunate prognosis, betrays no significant asphyxia to this baby. The absence of significant late, variable, or prolonged decelerations with induced contractions of this frequency in this chronically affected baby makes acute asphyxia implausible. At birth, the infant had Apgar scores of 5 and 8, nevertheless went on to have seizures in the neonatal period and at 6 months of age was found to have cerebral palsy.

REFERENCE

Shields JR, Schifrin BS: Perinatal antecedents of cerebral palsy. *Obstet Gynecol* 1988; 71:899.

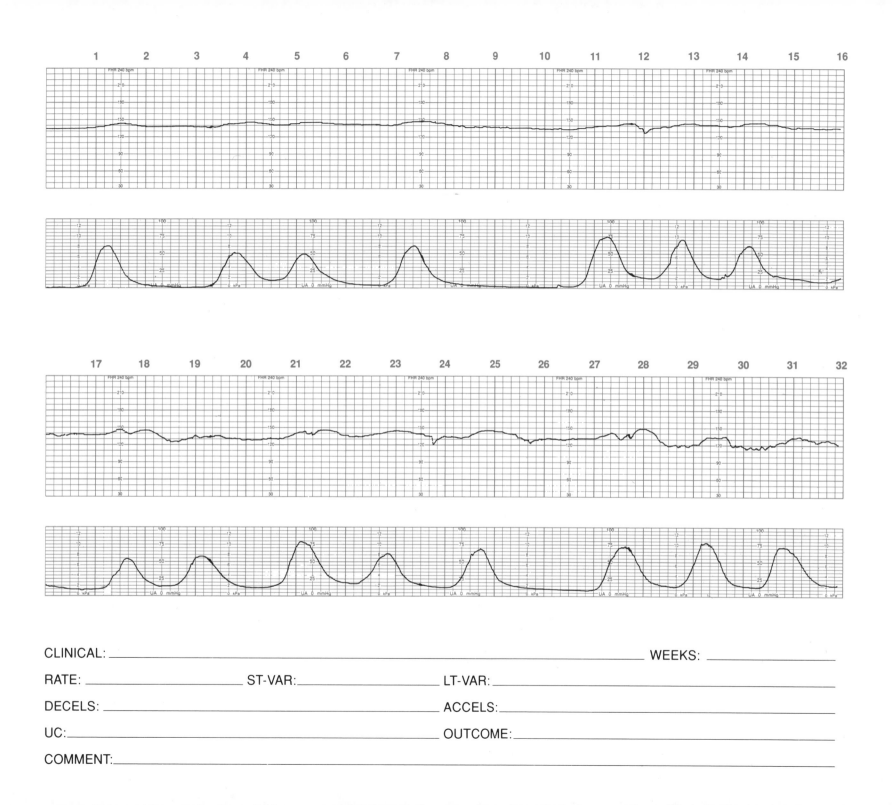

CLINICAL: _____ WEEKS: _____

RATE: _____ ST-VAR: _____ LT-VAR: _____

DECELS: _____ ACCELS: _____

UC: _____ OUTCOME: _____

COMMENT: _____

TRACING: 60

CLINICAL: IUGR.

WEEKS: 38

BASELINE RATE: 140

STV: Absent.

LTV: Decreased to absent.

DECELERATIONS: Variable.

ACCELERATIONS: Overshoot.

UC: Oxytocin.

OUTCOME: Cesarean section for failure to progress; Apgar scores 8/9; neonatal hypoglycemia; poor feeding; subsequent cerebral palsy.

COMMENT: This is another example of the chronic pattern. Baseline variability is markedly diminished, and the few recorded contractions elicit no decelerations. Small isolated variable decelerations (at 9M, 19M) occasionally punctuate the otherwise monotonous baseline. Added to the picture is one larger variable deceleration appearing during an episode of fetal arrhythmia which in turn provokes a brief episode of fetal bigeminy (at 25M). After several more ectopic beats, the arrhythmia resolves. As expected, the arrhythmia was not found after delivery. Along with the FHR pattern, the normal Apgar scores and absent acidosis preclude asphyxia during labor. The infant's only definable problems in the NICU were hypoglycemia and poor feeding. The infant subsequently developed cerebral palsy.

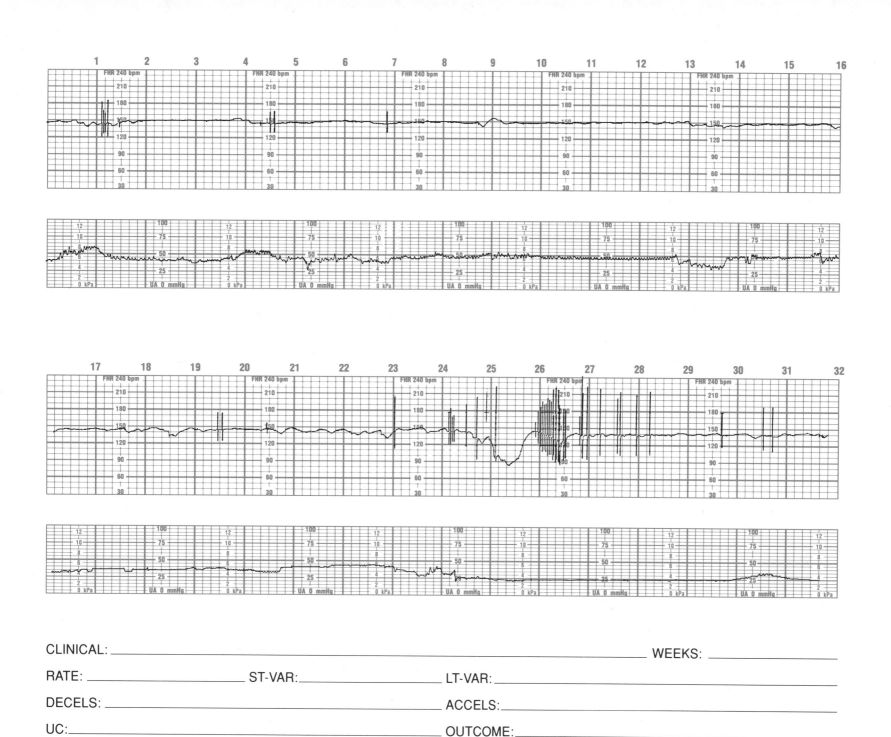

CLINICAL: _____ WEEKS: _____

RATE: _____ ST-VAR: _____ LT-VAR: _____

DECELS: _____ ACCELS: _____

UC: _____ OUTCOME: _____

COMMENT: _____

TRACING: 61

CLINICAL: Fetal maternal transfusion, NST.

WEEKS: 37

BASELINE RATE: 150

STV: Decreased.

LTV: Decreased.

DECELERATIONS: Mild variable.

ACCELERATIONS: None.

UC: None (NST).

OUTCOME: Neonatal hematocrit 11.5%.

COMMENT: This tracing reveals an intermittent sinusoidal pattern in an otherwise nearly flat baseline with mild variable decelerations. This pattern persisted despite vigorous attempts to stimulate the fetus. Absent drug effect or severe variable decelerations, this sinusoidal pattern is exemplary of fetal anemia (due to fetal maternal transfusion in this case) or Rh isoimmunization, although sepsis and cardiac anomaly must also be ruled out.

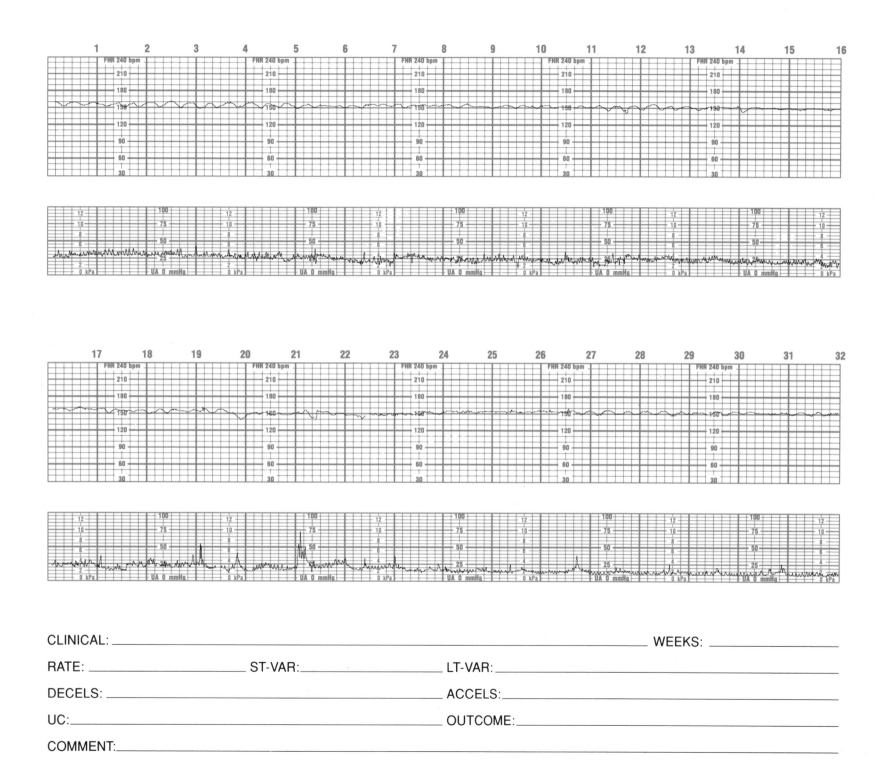

CLINICAL: _____ WEEKS: _____

RATE: _____ ST-VAR: _____ LT-VAR: _____

DECELS: _____ ACCELS: _____

UC: _____ OUTCOME: _____

COMMENT: _____

TRACING: 62

CLINICAL: Gestational diabetes.

WEEKS: 40

BASELINE RATE: Upper: 160   Lower: 130

STV: Decreased, absent.

LTV: Decreased, absent.

DECELERATIONS: Variable.

ACCELERATIONS: Overshoot.

UC: Irregular.

OUTCOME: Cesarean section; Apgar scores 1/0; 11-lb baby; peeling skin; meconium aspiration; neonatal death.

COMMENT: The *upper panel* shows the results of an NST (spontaneous CST) performed on this gestational diabetic patient at 40 weeks. The pattern is nonreactive with decreased variability and mild variable decelerations. In the labor suite shortly before delivery *(lower panel)* the pattern has degenerated to one of absent variability with variable decelerations. Uterine contractions are poorly recorded. In the final 4 minutes the falling baseline is punctuated by artifact, but seems to illustrate very regular high frequency, low amplitude oscillations incompatible with normal variability. This may represent the sawtooth pattern that is often associated with neurologic injury (see tracings 82, 83, 84). This baby was severely depressed and acidotic at the time of delivery, with cord pH 6.9 and neonatal base excess of −28 (see cord gases).

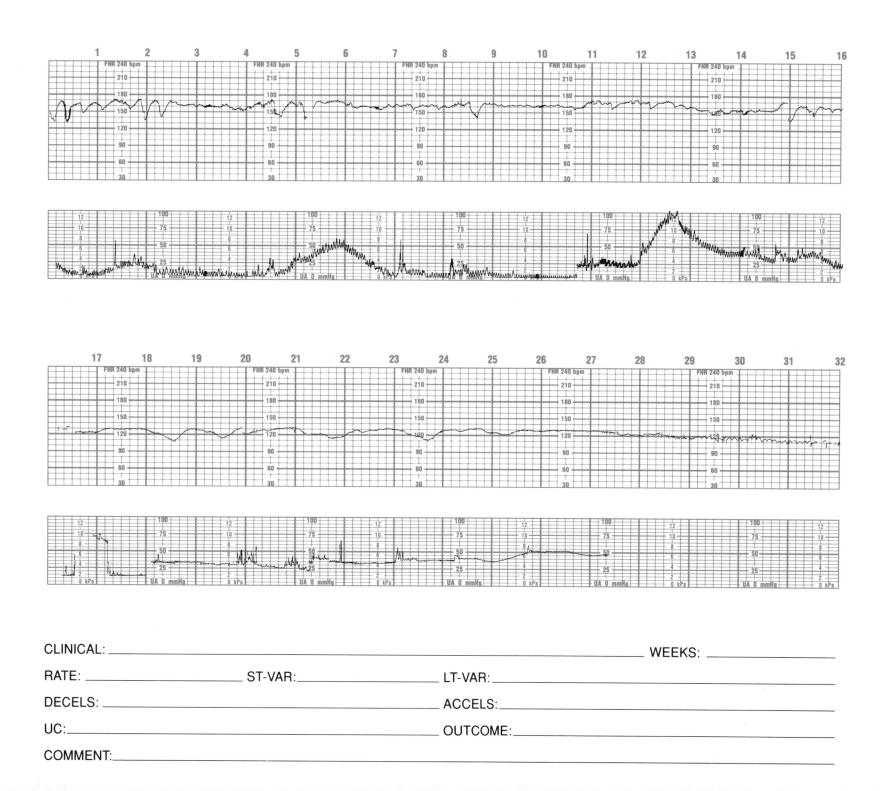

CLINICAL: _____ WEEKS: _____

RATE: _____ ST-VAR: _____ LT-VAR: _____

DECELS: _____ ACCELS: _____

UC: _____ OUTCOME: _____

COMMENT: _____

TRACING: 63

CLINICAL: Postdate pregnancy.

WEEKS: 41

RATE: 165–170

STV: Absent.

LTV: Absent, sinusoidal.

DECELERATION: Variable.

ACCELERATION: Absent.

UC: Frequent, irregular.

NST: Nonreactive.

CST: Negative.

OUTCOME: Apgar scores 2/6; neurologic handicap.

COMMENT: Although this tracing would qualify as a negative CST, suspicious to some, the combination of baseline tachycardia, nonreactive NST, and isolated, variable decelerations carries potentially ominous connotations. There are occasional maternal movements but no fetal movements. Except for the artifact between 13M and 15M, no excursion in the UC channel, whether it be maternal movements or UC, produces any response in FHR. In a normal, mature fetus, variable decelerations will elicit either the appearance of erratic accelerations (shoulders) or increased variability in the baseline after the deceleration. The fe-

tus may even become reactive—at least transiently. In this fetus, no such responses are forthcoming. Note the suggestion of sinusoidal pattern between 2M and 4M and perhaps after the deceleration as well.

When these features are seen in late pregnancy, the diagnosis of oligohydramnios or other source of cord compromise should be entertained and delivery expedited irrespective of the negative CST. In this case, ultrasound scanning revealed oligohydramnios and delivery was effected immediately. This meconium-stained, dysmature, nonasphyxiated infant received Apgar scores of 2 and 6 with normal cord pH values and had seizures within the first 24 hours of life. The infant subsequently demonstrated neurologic handicap.

142

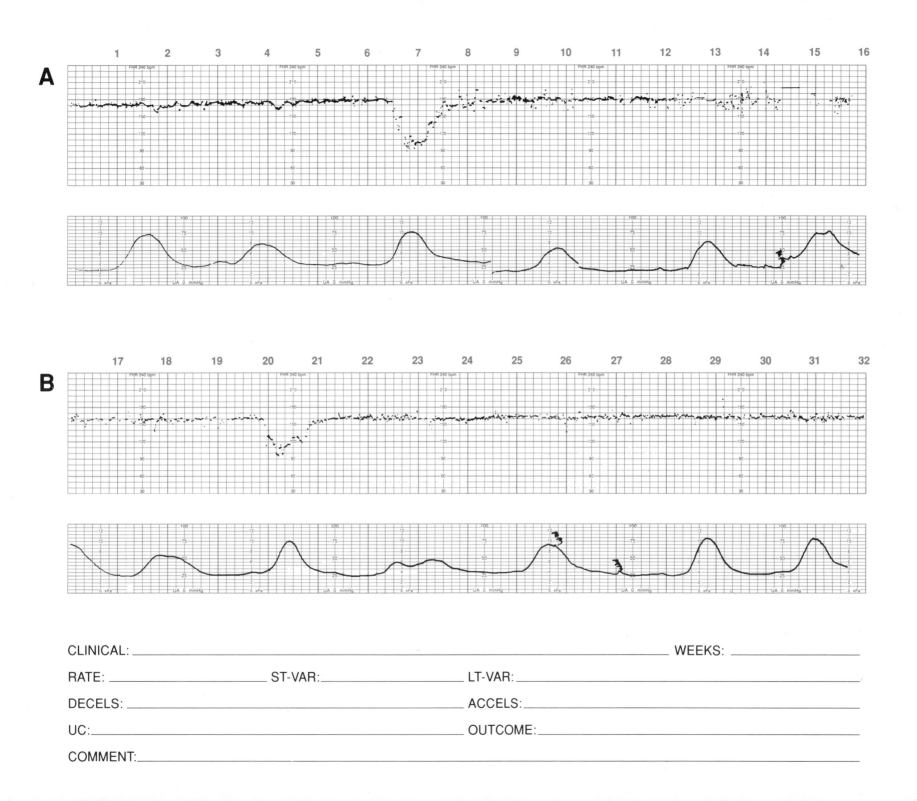

CLINICAL: _____ WEEKS: _____

RATE: _____ ST-VAR: _____ LT-VAR: _____

DECELS: _____ ACCELS: _____

UC: _____ OUTCOME: _____

COMMENT: _____

TRACING: 64

CLINICAL: Chorioamnionitis; labor.

WEEKS: 38

BASELINE RATE: 170

STV: Decreased.

LTV: Decreased.

DECELERATIONS: Variable.

ACCELERATIONS: Shoulders, overshoot.

UC: Increased resting tone.

OUTCOME: Apgar scores 5/7; apparently normal outcome.

COMMENT: This tracing bears some resemblance to the chronic pattern. It is introduced here to illustrate that certain clinical circumstances may conspire to produce a similar pattern in the absence of fetal injury or drug effect. The pattern of chronic distress really represents "impaired autonomic balance" with decreased parasympathetic tone compared with sympathetic tone. Thus prematurity, vagolytic drugs (e.g., atropine), and tachycardia of any cause (but especially fever) may simulate the chronic pattern. This tracing demonstrates an elevated baseline, decreased but not absent variability, and variable decelerations with overshoot. The artifact on the UC channel represents repeated efforts at changing the mother's position in attempts to relieve the decelerations. As the tracing continues, the variability continues to diminish and the decelerations continue to decrease in amplitude even in response to the more frequent uterine contractions.

The elevated fetal heart rate in this case represents a response to maternal pyrexia. It is unlikely that injury or asphyxia or even atropine will produce a heart rate in excess of 150 to 160 bpm. Unlike the decelerations associated with injury (e.g., tracings 43, 57, 58, 59), accelerations both precede and follow the decelerations.

Finally, the baseline appears, at least at the outset of the tracing, to maintain some variability. Though moderately depressed at delivery, this infant apparently survived intact.

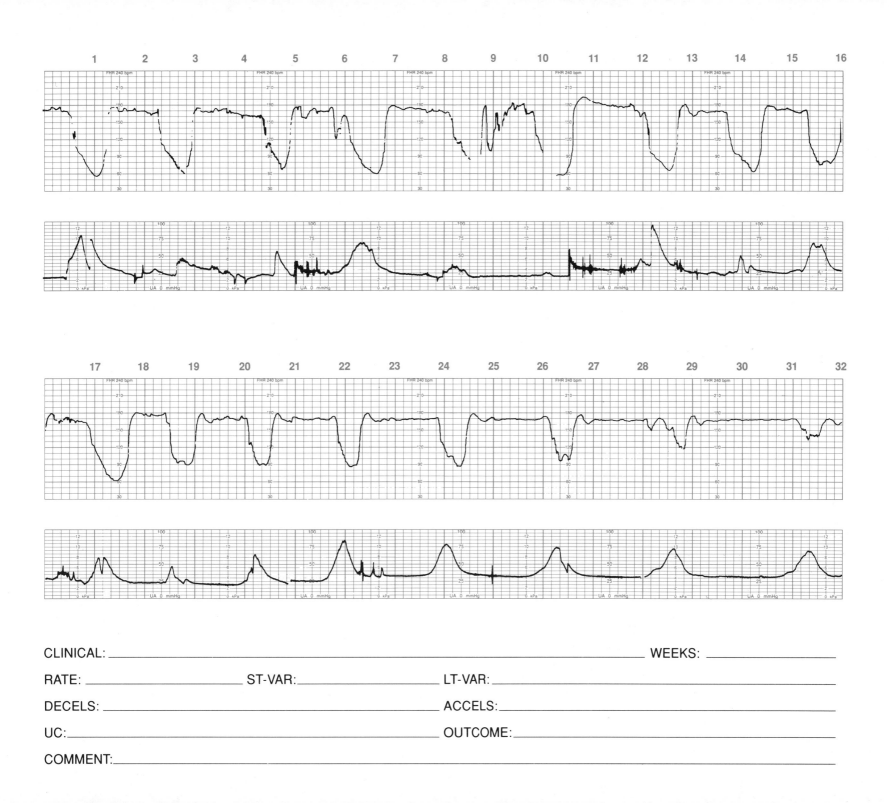

CLINICAL: _____ WEEKS: _____

RATE: _____ ST-VAR:_____ LT-VAR: _____

DECELS: _____ ACCELS:_____

UC:_____ OUTCOME:_____

COMMENT:_____

TRACING: 65

CLINICAL: NST, positive fetal movement,
biophysical profile = 10/12.

WEEKS: 42

BASELINE RATE: 160

STV: Decreased.

LTV: Absent.

DECELERATIONS: None.

ACCELERATIONS: None.

UC: Occasional.

OUTCOME: Vaginal delivery; Apgar scores 5/8;
shoulder dystocia.
Nursery: PAT, normal neonatal course.

COMMENT: This tracing was obtained in early labor at 42 weeks' gestation. The NST immediately preceding this tracing was nonreactive despite abundant fetal movement. A biophysical profile had revealed an active fetus with adequate amniotic fluid volume. This combination of an active fetus with a markedly abnormal FHR pattern should immediately suggest the possibility of an anomaly, neurologic abnormality, drugs, or arrhythmia. In this case, the explanation lies with an arrhythmia which was not detectable using an electronic device. Auscultation with an old-fashioned fetoscope would have revealed a heart rate approximately double that which the fetal monitor was recording. Because the monitor cannot record heart rates in excess of 210–240 bpm, it tends to half-count these rates. The individual beats in a PAT are notoriously regular, i.e., they produce absent variability.

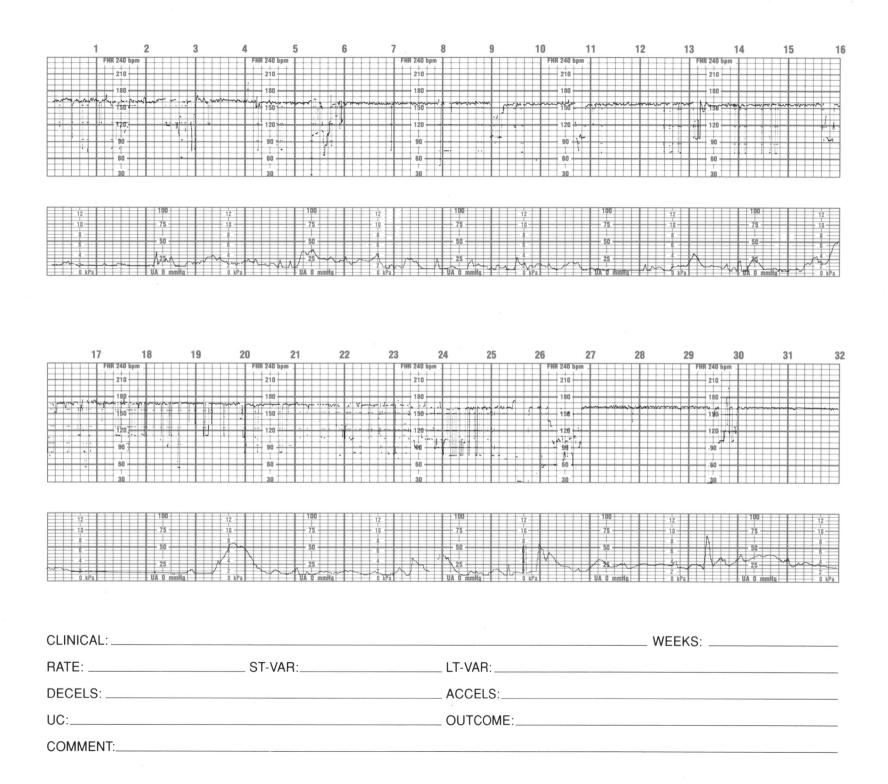

CLINICAL: _____ WEEKS: _____

RATE: _____ ST-VAR: _____ LT-VAR: _____

DECELS: _____ ACCELS: _____

UC: _____ OUTCOME: _____

COMMENT: _____

TRACING: 66

CLINICAL: Labor.

WEEKS: 37

BASELINE RATE: 110, unstable.

STV: Increased.

2LTV: Average.

DECELERATIONS: Present.

ACCELERATIONS: Coalesced, isolated.

UC: Irregular, early labor.

OUTCOME: Apgar scores 1/1; hydrocephalus; multiple anomalies; neonatal death.

COMMENT: This tracing reveals an unstable baseline, exaggerated short-term variability, and rather bizarre accelerations with uterine contractions, some of which coalesce. These unusual changes and excursions, as well as the instability of the overall rate, argue for an abnormal neurologic control over the heart rate. The fetus was known to be hydrocephalic and died shortly after birth with multiple anomalies.

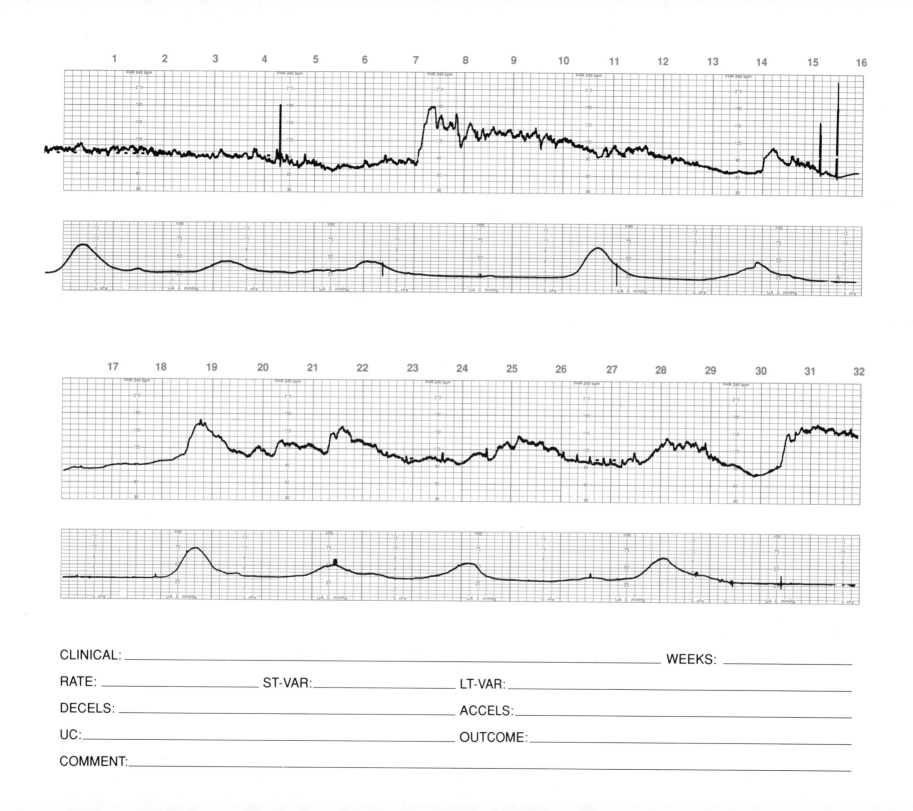

CLINICAL: _____ WEEKS: _____

RATE: _____ ST-VAR: _____ LT-VAR: _____

DECELS: _____ ACCELS: _____

UC: _____ OUTCOME: _____

COMMENT: _____

TRACING: 67

CLINICAL: IUGR, labor.

WEEKS: 38

BASELINE RATE: 155

STV: Probably decreased.

LTV: Decreased.

DECELERATIONS: Variable.

ACCELERATIONS: Suggestion of overshoot.

UC: Labor.

OUTCOME: Cesarean section; Apgar scores, 0, 0; CPR; baby lived 9 months; microcephalus; failure to thrive; anomalous syndrome.

COMMENT: This tracing derives from a patient who was in labor only a short time prior to emergency cesarean section. The heart rate pattern is abnormal from the very outset. The baseline heart rate exceeds 150–160 bpm and variable decelerations accompany virtually every contraction. The decelerations vary in amplitude from 50 bpm to almost 80 or 90 bpm and last between 45–50 seconds, although the last series lasts in excess of 4 minutes. Frequent decelerations and the high baseline are obvious, but the variability is probably decreased, though exaggerated by the ultrasound transducer. There is a small period of double counting at 27M. The return of the decelerations to baseline suggests overshoot or at least a rounded, smooth return.

Consistently, each downslope of the variable deceleration proceeds at a shallow angle in stepwise fashion. There is little to suggest that the baby deteriorates during the approximately 30 minutes of tracing available. Indeed, irrespective of the profound decelerations present, there is no dramatic shift in the baseline rate or change in the apparent variability. The fetus was delivered about 30 minutes after the end of the tracing. It was profoundly depressed, severely growth-retarded, and revealed obvious facial abnormalities.

Ultimately, the pattern is more consistent with anomaly than severe depression. Anomalous fetuses account for about 20% of abnormal antepartum FHR patterns. The patterns are occasionally bizarre or may simulate normal patterns or classic late or variable decelerations.

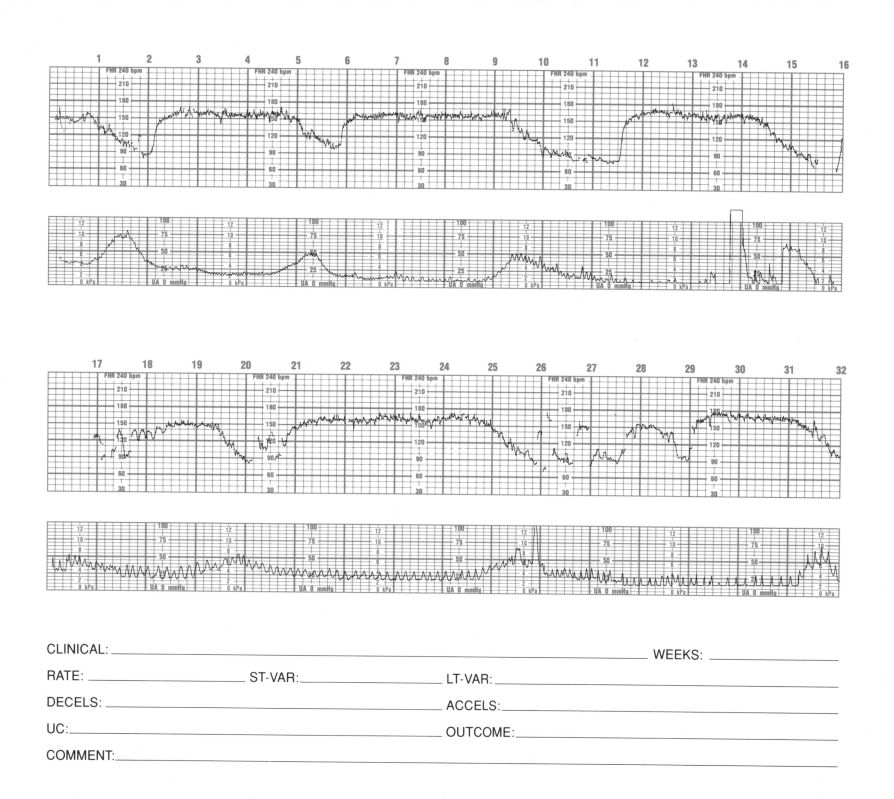

CLINICAL:_____ WEEKS:_____

RATE:_____ ST-VAR:_____ LT-VAR:_____

DECELS:_____ ACCELS:_____

UC:_____ OUTCOME:_____

COMMENT:_____

TRACING: 68

CLINICAL: Both: Known hydrocephalus

WEEKS: Upper: 32   Lower: 38

BASELINE RATE: Upper: 180   Lower: 130

STV: Both: Decreased.

LTV: Both: Absent.

DECELERATIONS: Upper: Variable. Lower: Prolonged, spontaneous.

ACCELERATIONS: Both: None.

UC: Labor.

OUTCOME: A: Apgar scores 0/0. B: Fetal death
during decompression procedure.

COMMENT: These two anomalous fetuses with known hydrocephalus illustrate markedly abnormal tracings. The patterns, nevertheless, are not diagnostic of anomaly, only of significant abnormality. The *upper panel* reveals baseline tachycardia, decreased variability, recurrent variable decelerations with overshoot—consistent with the chronic pattern. The *lower panel* begins with an average rate and at least long-term variability. The preceding tracing was unremarkable, even in the face of inserting a needle into the cerebral spinal fluid for decompression of the hydrocephalus. As the fluid was being removed, blood suddenly began to drain through the needle—a massive intracranial hemorrhage. Immediately upon the appearance of the hemorrhage, the fetal heart rate fell to 60 bpm, with markedly decreased variability. Shortly thereafter, the tracing was punctuated by dramatic accelerations. Then the fetal heart rate dropped further and the fetus died. This pattern is rather typical of massive fetal hemorrhage from anywhere, such as ruptured vasa praevia, whether the baby is anomalous or not. The pattern of acute hemorrhage should be separated from the sinusoidal pattern associated with the chronic anemia of Rh disease or maternal-fetal hemorrhage, and the appearance of late decelerations when blood loss is less acute.

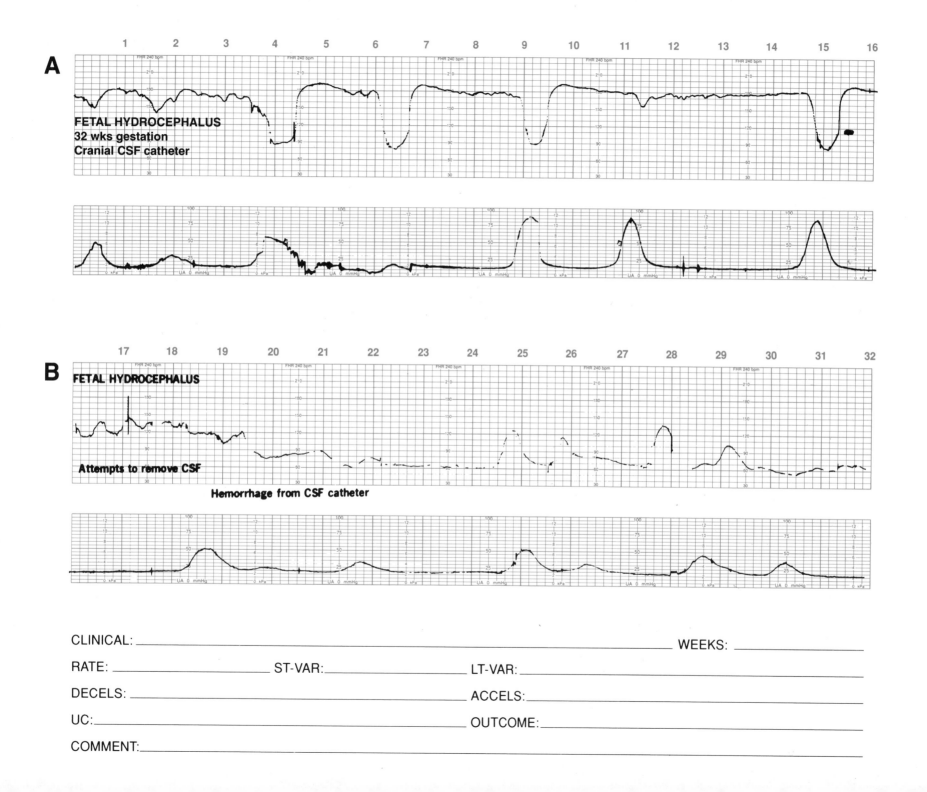

A

1 2 3 4 5 6 7 8 9 10 11 12 13 14 15 16

FETAL HYDROCEPHALUS
32 wks gestation
Cranial CSF catheter

B

17 18 19 20 21 22 23 24 25 26 27 28 29 30 31 32

FETAL HYDROCEPHALUS

Attempts to remove CSF

Hemorrhage from CSF catheter

CLINICAL: _____ WEEKS: _____

RATE: _____ ST-VAR: _____ LT-VAR: _____

DECELS: _____ ACCELS: _____

UC: _____ OUTCOME: _____

COMMENT: _____

TRACING: 69

CLINICAL: Polyhydramnios.

WEEKS: 34

RATE: Upper: 180   Lower: 120

STV: Absent.

LTV: Diminished.

DECELERATIONS: Variable.

ACCELERATIONS: Overshoot, unclassified (30M).

UC: Late labor.

OUTCOME: Multiple congenital anomalies incompatible with life.

COMMENT: This tracing and tracing 70 are offered here to startle and puzzle the reader. Even superficial inspection will reveal that the tracing is most abnormal. But is the baby asphyxiated? The tracing begins with a flat heart rate at 180 bpm, accompanied by usually small, variable decelerations with overshoot at 3M, 6M, 13M, and 14M. At 17M we find an abrupt descent to a stable rate of 120 bpm with equally diminished variability. From this new rate, usually small, variable decelerations with overshoot appear at 19M, 21M, and 25M. The overshoot after 25M defies description. It presents with an abrupt, angular upswing at 25M+ and a sudden transient downswing just after 26M. The same problem arises in the description of the acceleration(?) at 30M. The gradual rise is followed by an acute, right-angle deflection upward, then a slow decay and a right-angle deflection downward. Thus we have two separate heart rates, each stable, each giving off both abnormal or bizarre accelerations and decelerations.

Just as this sequence does not represent normal responsiveness, neither does it represent asphyxia. The presence of accelerations, the absence of repetitive decelerations, and the maintenance of a stable baseline rate all bespeak absent asphyxia. The abnormalities in the tracing are unique and do not subscribe to any normal definition of accelerations.

This fetus has multiple congenital anomalies involving both the heart and the central nervous system. The more bizarre the pattern and the more "mixed signals" it gives off, the more one should consider congenital anomaly in the differential diagnosis.

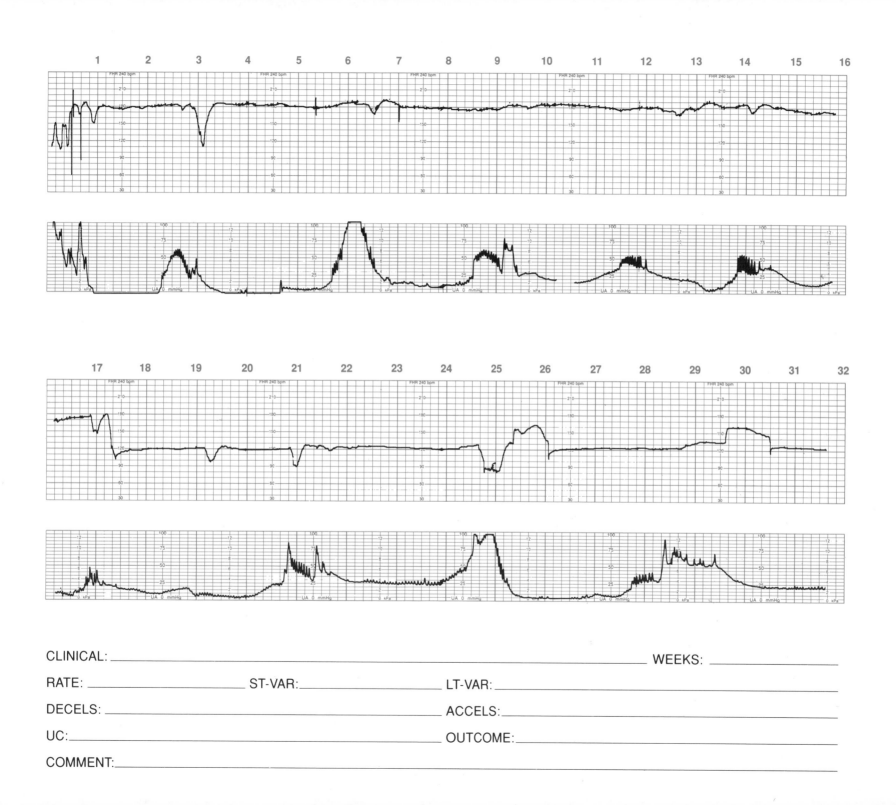

CLINICAL: _____ WEEKS: _____

RATE: _____ ST-VAR: _____ LT-VAR: _____

DECELS: _____ ACCELS: _____

UC: _____ OUTCOME: _____

COMMENT: _____

TRACING: 70

CLINICAL: Normal.

WEEKS: 37

BASELINE RATE: 160

STV: Absent.

LTV: Absent.

DECELERATIONS: Prolonged, variable.

ACCELERATIONS: Overshoot.

UC: Hypertonus.

OUTCOME: Normal.

COMMENT: This tracing reveals the effect of atropine injected directly into the fetus. At the outset, the baseline variability is normal and there are no decelerations. An increased frequency of uterine contractions and prolonged fetal deceleration accompanies the manipulation of the scalp necessary to inject the drug. This deceleration, nevertheless, retains a fair amount of variability. Upon completion of the injection there is a dramatic rise in the baseline to about 160 bpm. Even before the baseline heart rate has risen to its maximum level there is obvious diminution in the baseline variability. Indeed, loss of variability is the most consistent effect of atropine on the fetal or adult heart rate. Note also that provocation of the fetus (*between arrows*) produces small, irregularly shaped variable decelerations with overshoot.

While atropine is very rarely used, this tracing is inserted here to illustrate that the administration of autonomic drugs, in this case atropine, will mimic in virtually all respects the heart rate tracing associated with anomaly or injury. Atropine represents the pharmacologic impairment of the parasympathetic nervous system, the primary factor controlling the fetal cardiac variability and heart rate. It is thus most reasonable to refer to this pattern as impaired autonomic balance whose etiology may represent injury, anomaly, or medication, but which does not in and of itself represent fetal asphyxia. The most reliable and consistent effect of atropine is the reduction in baseline variability. Fetal tachycardia after atropine rarely exceeds 155 or 160 bpm. This response is also proportional to the resting baseline heart rate, i.e., the lower the baseline rate, the greater the response to atropine, and the higher the baseline rate, the less the response to atropine. Atropine may also uncover accelerations with contractions (see Tracing 69) and the telltale appearance of overshoot with the variable decelerations.

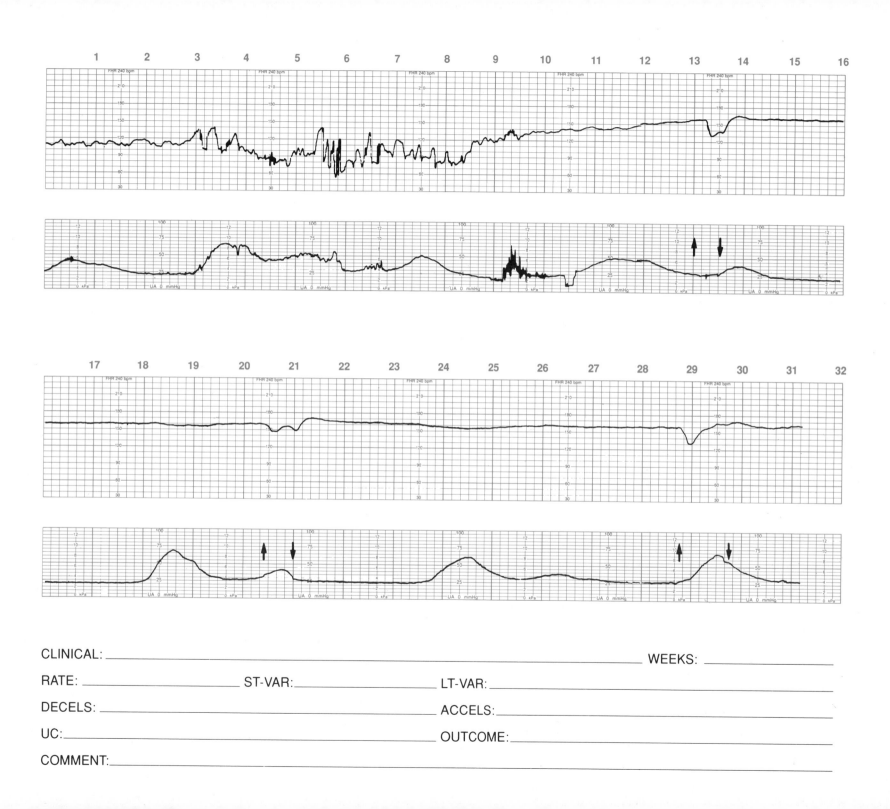

CLINICAL: _____ WEEKS: _____

RATE: _____ ST-VAR: _____ LT-VAR: _____

DECELS: _____ ACCELS: _____

UC: _____ OUTCOME: _____

COMMENT: _____

TRACING: 71

CLINICAL: Irregular heart beats.

WEEKS: Both: 38

RATE: A: 140   B: Your choice—140 or 170

STV: A: Decreased. B: Average.

LTV: A: Decreased. B: Decreased.

DECELERATIONS: A: Late. B: Variable.

ACCELERATIONS: A: Absent. B: Absent.

UC: A: Irregular. B: Regular, early labor.

NST: A: Nonreactive B: Nonreactive.

CST: A: Positive. B: Negative.

OUTCOME: A: IUGR; low Apgar scores. B: Heart block, normal.

COMMENT: The *upper panel* illustrates some technical difficulties in both heart rate and UC recording. The baseline fetal heart rate can only be estimated after some 7 or 8 minutes of tracing when the recurrent late decelerations become manifest. Decelerations are clearly present before that time, but because of the amplitude of the decelerations, the external ultrasound device doubles the fetal heart rate, creating a physiologically implausible pattern. Thus, the tracing segments between 3M and 4M and between 6M and 7M are artifact—the double-counted nadir of the late decelerations. The UC channel reveals recurrent obvious contractions which, at the beginning, are not well recorded although they can be inferred. This is a positive CST.

In the *lower panel,* obtained during labor, the true baseline rate cannot reasonably be ascertained without some insight. The most reasonable heart rate, about 140 bpm, alternates with transiently elevated heart rates at about 170–180 bpm. This sudden change in the rate, unlike the *upper panel,* represents intermittent PAT in a near-term fetus during labor. Note the stable rate preceding the transient jump in the heart rate at approximately 22M and just after 25M and the decay into the elevated rate of about 170–180 bpm. A single prolonged interval suddenly terminates the PAT episode. The acceleration (28M) and variable deceleration (30M) only occur with the lower rate which represents sinus rhythm. The abrupt changes in the rate here are not multiples of one another. They subscribe to a consistent pattern and are unlikely to represent miscounting or artifact. A direct electrocardiogram would provide evidence for the arrhythmia. Auscultation in both cases would clearly reveal the correct interpretation.

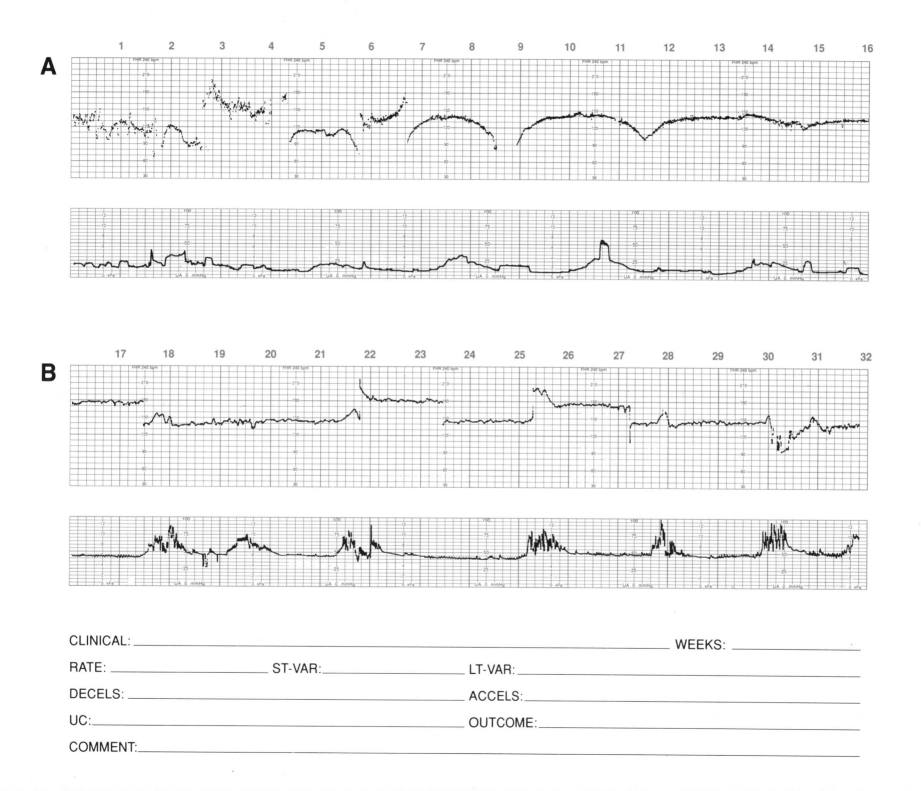

CLINICAL: _____   WEEKS: _____

RATE: _____ ST-VAR: _____ LT-VAR: _____

DECELS: _____ ACCELS: _____

UC: _____ OUTCOME: _____

COMMENT: _____

TRACING: 72

CLINICAL: Irregular heart beat.

WEEKS: 38

RATE: A: About 180   B: Mother, 90; fetus, 130

STV: A: Absent. B: Mother and fetus, average.

LTV: A: Absent. B: Mother and fetus, average.

DECELERATIONS: Both: Absent.

ACCELERATIONS: A: Absent. B: Sporadic.

UC: A: Frequent, oxytocin. B: Absent.

NST: A: Nonreactive. B: Reactive.

CST: A: Negative. B: Unsatisfactory.

OUTCOME: Both: Normal.

COMMENT: These two panels illustrate the potential confusion that may result from technical limitations of external monitoring techniques. Each technique for obtaining the fetal heart rate (internal or external) has the capability of misrepresenting both the rate and the variability. In the *upper panel,* this baby with PAT shows a heart rate of about 180 bpm. When the heart rate exceeds 180 bpm, the monitor will half-count and does so between 4M and 9M and from 13M on. These abrupt changes do not represent conversion or modification of the block but the difficulties in registering rapid heart rates with external devices. PAT patterns tend to be quite regular and show no influence from contractions or fetal movement. This finding should prompt ultrasound evaluation to ascertain the presence of either a cardiac anomaly or evidence of fetal ascites (heart failure).

The *lower panel* reveals an abrupt change in both the rate and reactivity. In this case it is the mother's heart rate that is being monitored between 16M and 21M. The mother's pattern, like the normal baby's, possesses some variability and is stable. The reactive tracing that appears from 22M on is sufficient to suggest that the preceding tracing is unrelated to the fetal condition.

In both *upper* and *lower panels,* a proper interpretation will be facilitated by either auscultation or by simultaneously monitoring the maternal heart rate. Some fetal monitors have the potential for recording both maternal and fetal heart rates simultaneously, and this should be performed on a regular basis. When such devices are unavailable, simultaneous monitoring with two separate fetal instruments should be employed. As with the monitoring of twins, both strips should be annotated simultaneously. When removed from the monitors, the two strips can be lined up to ascertain any differences in the two heart rate patterns.

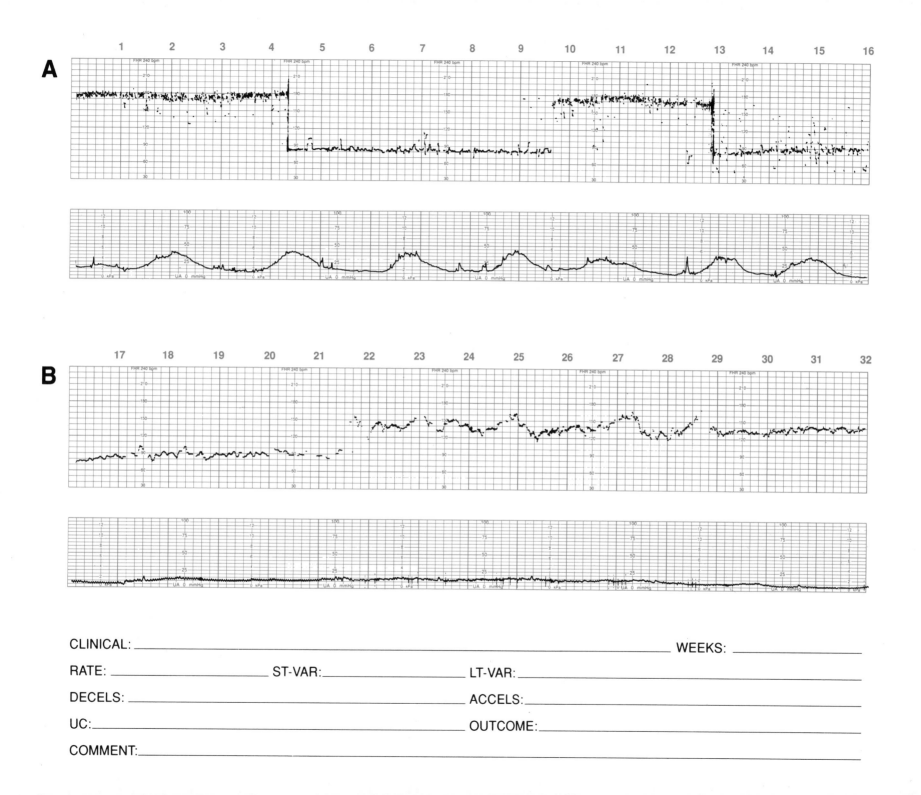

CLINICAL: _____   WEEKS: _____

RATE: _____ ST-VAR: _____ LT-VAR: _____

DECELS: _____   ACCELS: _____

UC: _____   OUTCOME: _____

COMMENT: _____

TRACING: 73

CLINICAL: A: Irregular heartbeat. B: Fetal death.

WEEKS: A: 41   B: 37

BASELINE RATE: A: 90, 170   B: 70, 210

STV: A: Average. B: Average.

LTV: A: Exaggerated. B: Average.

DECELERATIONS: A: None. B: None.

ACCELERATIONS: A: None. B: None.

UC: A: Latent phase. B: Labor.

OUTCOME: A: Normal. B: Stillbirth.

COMMENT: Panel A illustrates markedly exaggerated baseline variability associated with apparent baseline bradycardia in the few instances where baseline can be discerned. Such exaggerated variability is referred to as saltatory or as "vagal patterns," and while invariably benign, usually prompts concern for the well-being of the fetus. These patterns are most often seen after variable decelerations in the second stage of labor. They are especially common when the mother is unmedicated during labor. They appear to represent a dominance of vagal activity in the heart rate and fetal maturity as well. In other instances saltatory patterns may be seen to be less dramatic following the administration of ephedrine (see tracing 47).

The tracing in the *lower panel* represents a pattern obtained by a scalp electrode on a dead fetus. The totally random excursions with the constant low baseline heart rate in fact represent the counting of the maternal heart rate. Because of the low amplitude of the maternal signal, which is obtained through the dead fetus, the amplification must be extreme, and the greater the amplification of the signal, the greater the potential noise and artifact.

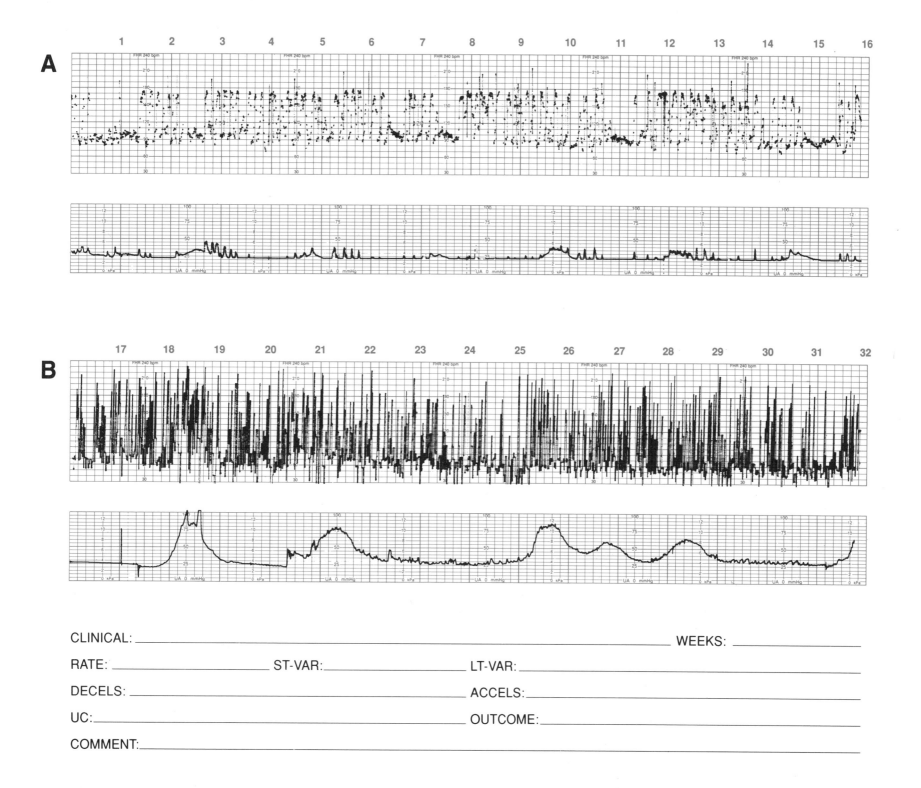

CLINICAL: _____ WEEKS: _____

RATE: _____ ST-VAR: _____ LT-VAR: _____

DECELS: _____ ACCELS: _____

UC: _____ OUTCOME: _____

COMMENT: _____

TRACING: 74

CLINICAL: Unremarkable prenatal course.

WEEKS: 42

BASELINE RATE: 180, 130, 110

STV: Decreased.

LTV: Decreased.

DECELERATIONS: None.

ACCELERATIONS: None.

UC: A: Advanced labor. B: Fetal ECG tracing.

OUTCOME: Apgar scores 8/9; no cardiac abnormality; persistent neonatal arrhythmia.

COMMENT: The *upper tracing* illustrates a reactive fetus that suddenly develops multiple supraventricular ectopic beats. Without warning at 8M the fetus develops supraventricular tachycardia (PAT) with a high degree of block. Equally abruptly the paroxysm breaks at 13M and with only an occasional ectopic beat the fetus resumes its normal pattern. There is no obvious relationship between the paroxysms and uterine contractions. Simultaneous recordings of fetal heart rate and fetal ECG during labor permit accurate diagnosis of this apparently benign arrhythmia. Neonatal heart rate and ECG recordings were identical to those obtained in utero.

The potential for recording the fetal ECG is illustrated in the *lower panel.* The fetal ECG written at 25 mm/sec replaces the UC channel. This heart rate was discovered by fetal heart auscultation 1½ hours after admission. Note the runs of bigeminal rhythm—ectopic beats alternating with normal ones—revealed by the opaque geometric blocks. This is identical to the pattern between 8M and 12M and contrasts with the block of similar breadth at 6M, which has a consistent mark above the midpoint. This represents trigeminy or quadrigeminy in which one ectopic beat alternates with two or three normal beats. Note the reproducible spikes in the heart rate at 18M, 19M, 20M, etc., which represent paroxysms of supraventricular tachycardia. The ECG pattern clearly illustrates both the bigeminy and the paroxysms. In both fetuses the ectopic beats were found in the neonatal period.

REFERENCE

Klapholz M, Schifrin BS, Rivo E: Paroxysmal supraventricular tachycardia in the fetus. *Obstet Gynecol* 1974; 43:718–721.

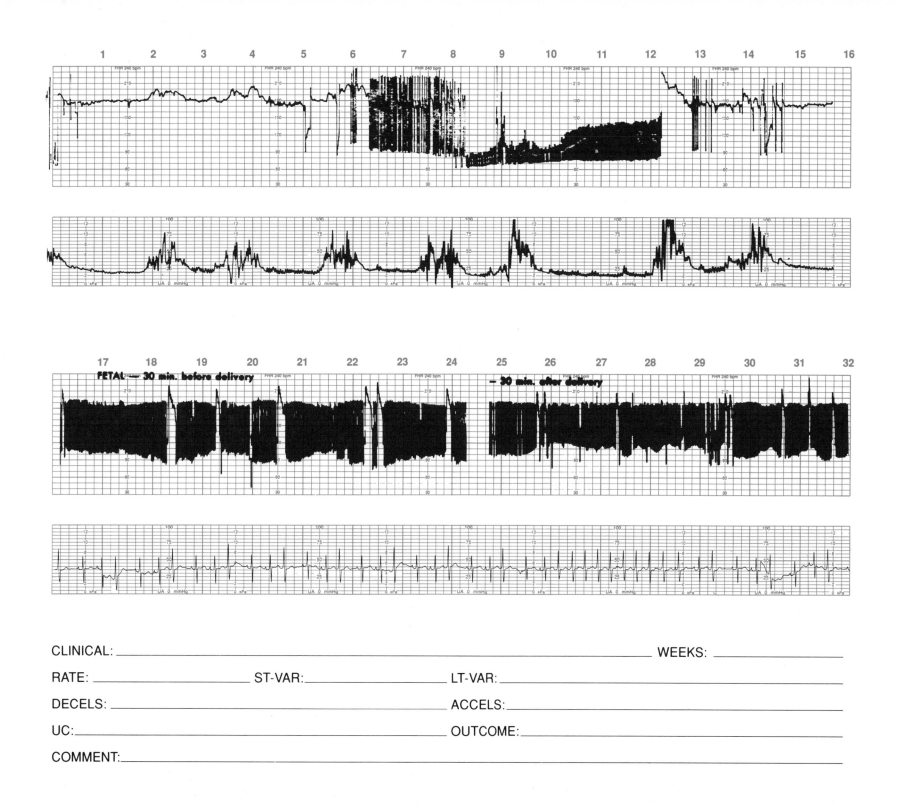

CLINICAL: _____ WEEKS: _____

RATE: _____ ST-VAR: _____ LT-VAR: _____

DECELS: _____ ACCELS: _____

UC: _____ OUTCOME: _____

COMMENT: _____

TRACING: 75

CLINICAL: Labor.

WEEKS: 37

BASELINE RATE: 120–130

STV: Average.

LTV: Average.

DECELERATIONS: Upper: None. Lower: Prolonged.

ACCELERATIONS: Upper: Reactive. Lower: None.

UC: Irregular.

OUTCOME: Apgar scores 5/8; neurologic injury.

COMMENT: This tracing and the one following illustrate the development of fetal neurologic injury during labor. The *upper panel* illustrates normal fetal reactivity with accelerations associated with fetal movement and average variability. In the *lower panel* several episodes of polysystole induce prolonged decelerations. The fetus seems to be recovering from the first deceleration at 21M, but the technical inadequacy of the tracing limits this conclusion. Just before the end of the tracing the fetus sustains a second prolonged deceleration. The recovery is depicted in the next tracing.

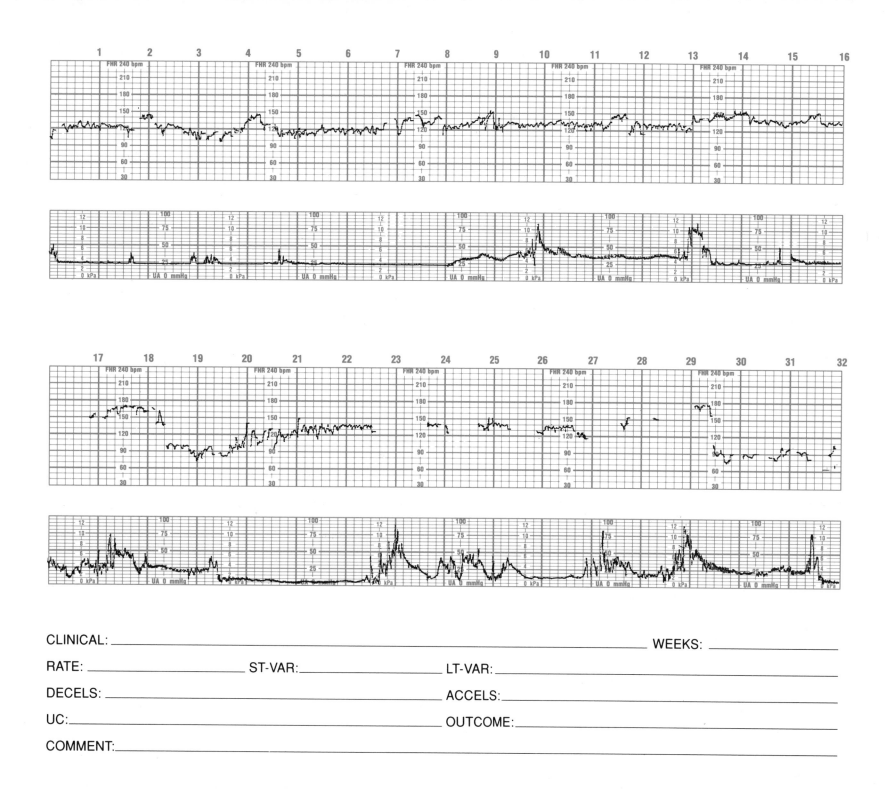

CLINICAL: _____ WEEKS: _____

RATE: _____ ST-VAR: _____ LT-VAR: _____

DECELS: _____ ACCELS: _____

UC: _____ OUTCOME: _____

COMMENT: _____

TRACING: 76

CLINICAL: Upper: Fetal scalp electrode. Lower: Second-stage labor.

WEEKS: 37

BASELINE RATE: 140–150

STV: Average to increased.

LTV: Upper: Decreased. Lower: Average, saltatory.

DECELERATIONS: Variable.

ACCELERATIONS: Upper: Absent. Lower: Sporadic.

UC: Upper: Coupling. Lower: Second stage.

OUTCOME: Apgar scores 5/8; cerebral palsy.

COMMENT: This tracing follows from tracing 75. After the prolonged decelerations and loss of signal, a fetal scalp electrode is applied *(upper panel)* revealing a flat baseline of 160 bpm, mild variable decelerations, and obvious high frequency, low amplitude oscillations. These should not be confused with variability. Note that the fetus still responds with early or variable (not late) decelerations and that there is no significant tachycardia.

The *lower panel* reflects the same fetus during the second stage of labor when still a fourth pattern emerges. This tracing shows an erratic saltatory pattern, at times with many variable decelerations and long-term variability, as long as the patient is pushing and contractions are close together. When the contrac-tions space out (28M), variability appears decreased and tiny accelerations punctuate the baseline.

This fetus is not asphyxiated, but the pattern following the period of prolonged decelerations could not be more divergent from the original reactive tracing and represents the recovery of an injured fetus. This is not true recovery but reestablishment of a heart rate and new pattern in a neurologically injured, nonasphyxiated fetus. The injury is sustained sometime after the original reactive tracing is recorded and before the *upper panel* on this page, reasonably during the prolonged decelerations, with the exact cause unknown.

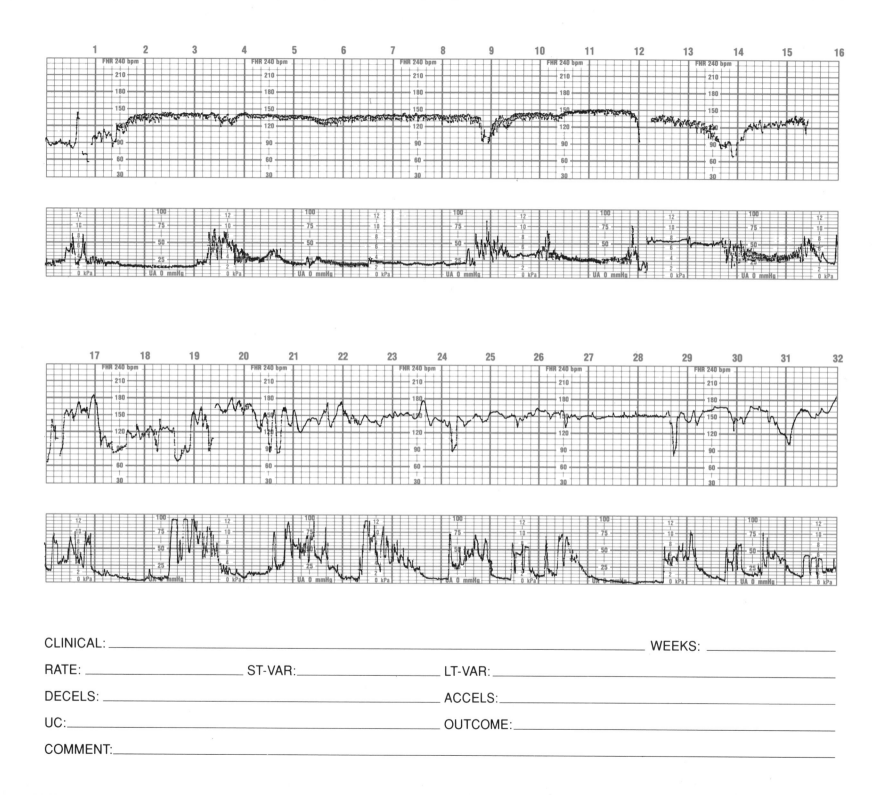

CLINICAL: _____ WEEKS: _____

RATE: _____ ST-VAR: _____ LT-VAR: _____

DECELS: _____ ACCELS: _____

UC: _____ OUTCOME: _____

COMMENT: _____

TRACING: 77

CLINICAL: PIH; meconium; meperidine; oxytocin.

WEEKS: 43+

BASELINE RATE: 160

STV: Exaggerated.

LTV: Exaggerated.

DECELERATIONS: None.

ACCELERATIONS: Coalesced.

UC: Oxytocin.

OUTCOME: Maternal seizure; cesarean section;
Apgar scores 2/4/5; fetal macrosomia; meconium aspiration;
living neonate; cerebral palsy.

COMMENT: This tracing reveals exaggerated (saltatory) long-term variability that at times coalesces to form the oddly geometric-looking decelerations associated with the maternal bearing-down efforts on the *lower tracing.* This mother has severe PIH untreated except for narcotics. Her elevated blood pressure is exacerbated by very frequent oxytocin-induced contractions and frequent bearing-down efforts. The exaggerated variability seems to reflect a vagal effect from the bearing-down efforts. At least on the *upper panel,* the variability between contractions is less dramatic. The decelerations likely represent fetal nodal rhythm—another manifestation of the enhanced vagal tone. They do not comport with late decelerations or obvious asphyxial fetal distress. At the end of the tracing the mother has a seizure and the fetal heart rate begins to fall. Moderation of the oxytocin infusion rate and administration of $MgSO_4$ should have been undertaken before the situation reached this point. The tracing is continued on tracing 78.

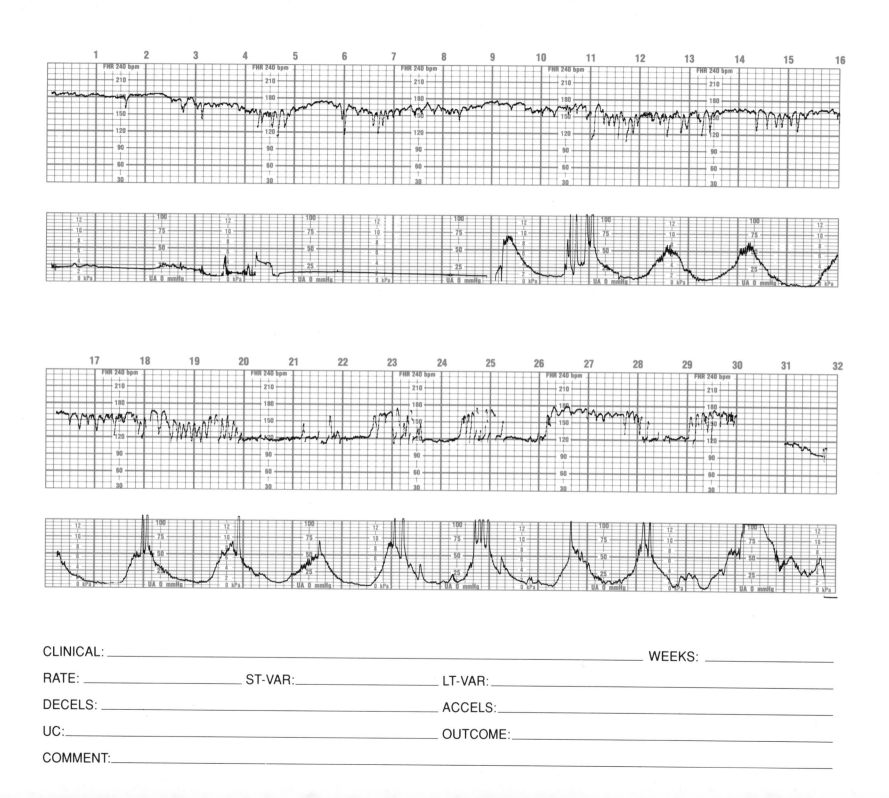

CLINICAL: _____ WEEKS: _____

RATE: _____ ST-VAR: _____ LT-VAR: _____

DECELS: _____ ACCELS: _____

UC: _____ OUTCOME: _____

COMMENT: _____

TRACING: 78

CLINICAL: PIH; maternal seizure; $MgSO_4$.

WEEKS: 42+

BASELINE RATE: 180

STV: Absent.

LTV: Absent.

DECELERATIONS: Prolonged.

ACCELERATIONS: None.

UC: None or not recorded.

OUTCOME: Cesarean section; Apgar scores 2/4; cerebral palsy.

COMMENT: This tracing is derived from the same patient as tracing 77. In the *upper panel* the mother has had an eclamptic seizure and has been given barbiturates as well as $MgSO_4$. The fetus has sustained a prolonged bradycardia to 60 bpm and is slowly recovering. The pattern eventually proceeds to a compensatory tachycardia of 180 bpm with absent variability and the suggestion of the curious small acceleration-deceleration complexes at 9M+, 11M, and 14M+. The *lower panel* shows a ruler-flat, sometimes sinusoidal baseline of 175 bpm. Shortly thereafter the baby was delivered. Although some of the diminu-tion is attributable to drug effect, this baby is clearly injured during the maternal seizure and goes on to manifest neurologic injury. The scalp pH obtained near the end of the *upper panel* was 7.0 and a cesarean section was performed. This confirmed the obvious asphyxial episode but unfortunately was not repeated to illustrate the probable recovery. A cord pH at the time of delivery 30 minutes later showed only mild metabolic acidosis. The infant suffered seizures in the neonatal nursery and was later diagnosed as having cerebral palsy.

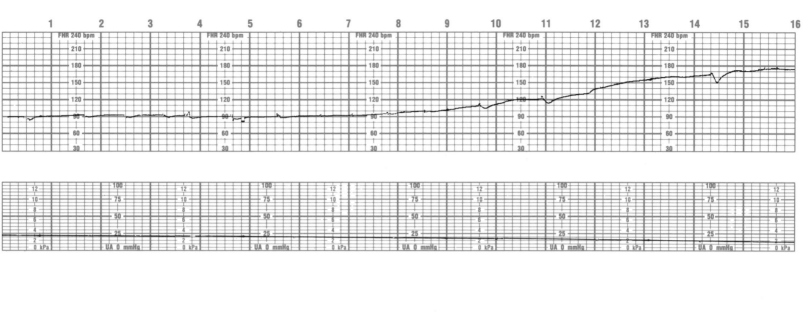

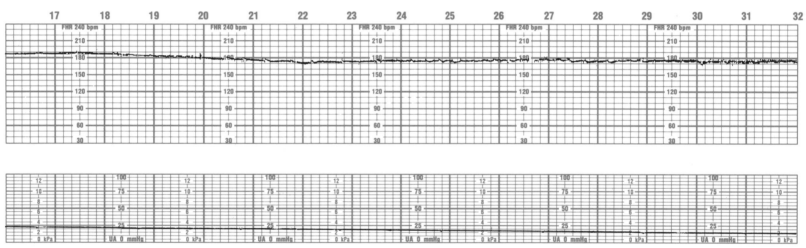

CLINICAL: _____ WEEKS: _____

RATE: _____ ST-VAR: _____ LT-VAR: _____

DECELS: _____ ACCELS: _____

UC: _____ OUTCOME: _____

COMMENT: _____

TRACING: 79

CLINICAL: Uneventful pregnancy

WEEKS: 40

BASELINE RATE: 140

STV: Decreased

LTV: Decreased

DECELERATIONS: Prolonged.

ACCELERATIONS: Bizarre.

UC: Frequent.

OUTCOME: Apgar scores 1/3; neurologic injury.

COMMENT: This tracing illustrates the development of fetal injury following paracervical block using 0.5% bupivacaine injection. At the outset, the baseline heart rate is quite stable. There are no decelerations, and variability, though somewhat decreased owing to maternal medication, is otherwise reassuring. Just prior to the onset of the *lower panel,* the patient was given 10 mL of 0.5% bupivacaine on each side as a paracervical block. This precipitated, though poorly recorded, very frequent uterine contractions and fetal bradycardia. The deceleration lasted about 7 minutes and appeared to be recovering when the heart rate suddenly plummeted to 60 bpm, with absent variability. The tracing is then punctuated only by brief, aberrant acceleration-deceleration complexes associated with intermittent attempts at stimulating the fetus through the abdomen. While this stimulation appears to provoke these curious accelerations, it had no impact on either the sustained bradycardia or the absent variability.

The mechanism of this change, though unclear, would seem to be involved with the circulation and uptake of this potentially toxic local anesthetic into the fetal circulation. It should be emphasized that the appearance of bradycardia, unrelated to excessive uterine activity, suggests that the fetus received an intoxicating amount of drug. This infant was born markedly depressed and has residual neurologic deficit. It seems reasonable to say that this injury was related to the administration of paracervical block. While there is markedly decreased use of paracervical block today, it remains a quite safe technique provided proper attention is paid to the drug, the dosage, and fetal well-being prior to administration of the drug. Under no circumstances should bupivacaine be used.

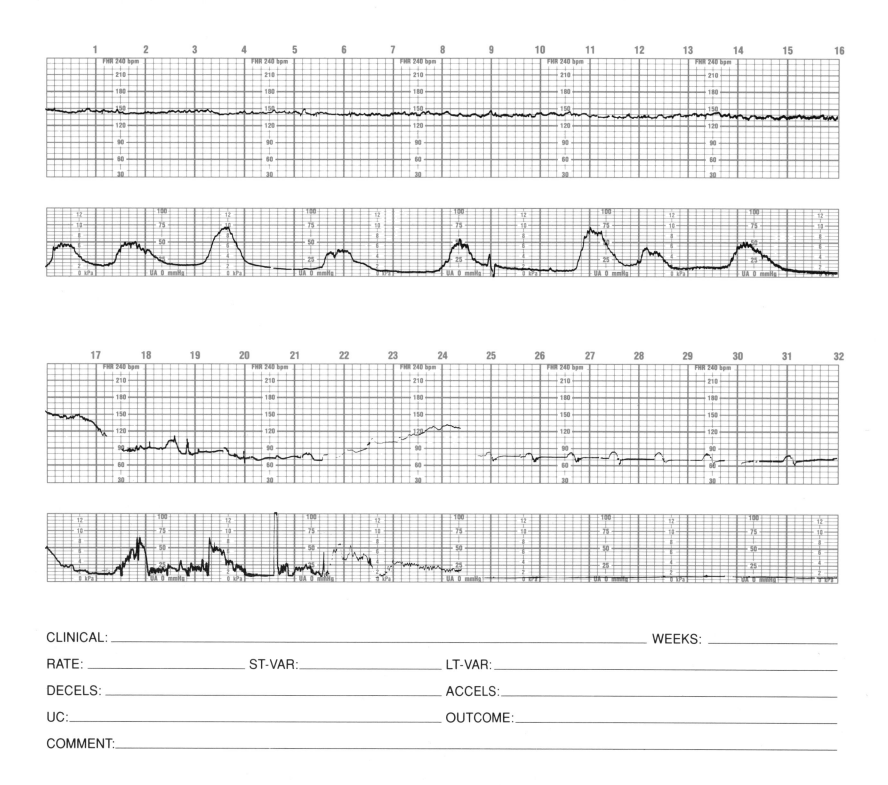

CLINICAL: _____ WEEKS: _____

RATE: _____ ST-VAR: _____ LT-VAR: _____

DECELS: _____ ACCELS: _____

UC: _____ OUTCOME: _____

COMMENT: _____

TRACING: 80

CLINICAL: Prolonged labor, OP position.

WEEKS: 40

BASELINE RATE: 140

STV: Average.

LTV: Average.

DECELERATIONS: Variable.

ACCELERATIONS: Sporadic.

UC: IUPC

OUTCOME: Apgar scores 2/4/5.

COMMENT: This tracing is provided in several parts to illustrate the unusual evolution of a fetus with a normal heart rate pattern evolving into injury during the second stage of labor, probably related to the combination of bearing-down efforts and the marked molding associated with OP position. The tracing begins normally enough with a baseline of about 140 bpm, average variability, accelerations, and few periodic changes with uterine contractions. The *lower panel* reveals increasing variability and greater excursions as the frequency of contractions increases and bearing-down efforts begin. This tracing is reasonably reassuring and requires no treatment. Please proceed to tracing 81.

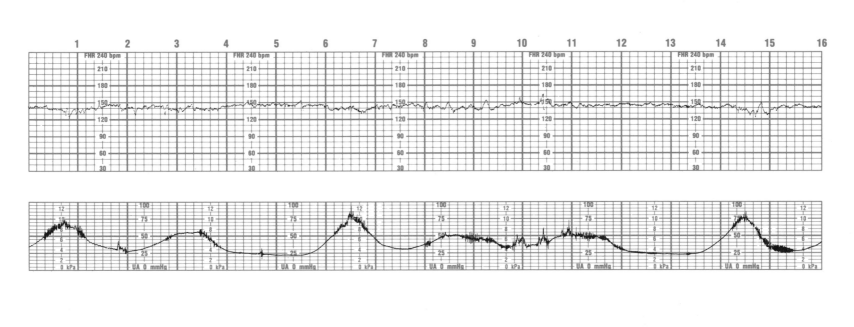

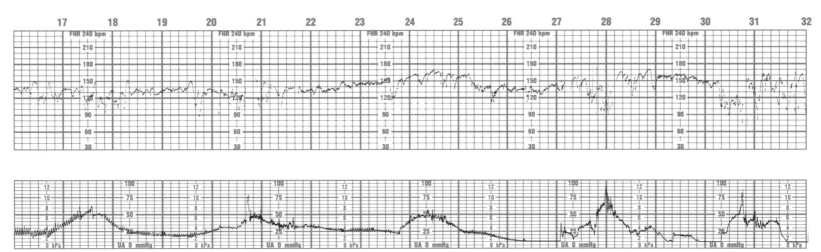

CLINICAL: _____ WEEKS: _____

RATE: _____ ST-VAR: _____ LT-VAR: _____

DECELS: _____ ACCELS: _____

UC: _____ OUTCOME: _____

COMMENT: _____

TRACING: 81

CLINICAL: Prolonged labor, OP position.

WEEKS: 40

BASELINE RATE: 120, rising thereafter.

STV: Average, increased, absent.

LTV: Average, increased, absent.

DECELERATIONS: Mild variable.

ACCELERATIONS: None.

UC: Bearing down.

OUTCOME: Apgar scores 2/4/5; neonatal seizures; intracranial hemorrhage.

COMMENT: These panels are continued from tracing 80. Note that the baseline heart rate is now less than 120 bpm. This represents a small but significant drop in the baseline heart rate associated with an increase in the baseline variability. This pattern, while normal and seen without the benefit of the preceding tracing, would cause little concern. More detailed analysis suggests that it represents the effects of fetal hypertension and increased intracranial pressure related to the frequent contractions, the almost continuous expulsive efforts, and perhaps the marked molding in the OP position. Note the apparent attempt at recovery when the pushing is diminished at 9M. At 9 minutes the pattern changes dramatically. Initially the rate is now about 140 bpm, variability is somewhat decreased, and there are isolated, discrete variable decelerations. In the *lower panel* the baseline heart rate has risen to 170 bpm and despite some considerable artifact, the baseline variability is now totally absent. Despite the almost constant pushing and further descent of the fetal head to the point of delivery, there are now no decelerations and the variability could not be flatter. Upon delivery from the OP position, the infant was found to be markedly depressed and shortly thereafter had a seizure. Evaluation revealed significant intracranial hemorrhage.

It seems reasonable to infer that the injury began at about 9M on the *top panel* where the dramatic change first appears. It appears that its evolution is complete by the end of the tracing. Though this dramatic event was neither predictable nor related to any deficiency in the quality of the care offered the patient, several conclusions may be inferred: the mechanical effects from expulsion, position, or molding of the head may indeed contribute to the development of injury irrespective of the quality of medical care. It further suggests perhaps several clinical strategies: (1) Awareness that a low baseline, despite its normal variability, may in fact represent a baby that is already compensating, and (2) efforts should be made in cases such as this to diminish the amount and frequency of the expulsive efforts, perhaps limiting pushing efforts to every other contraction.

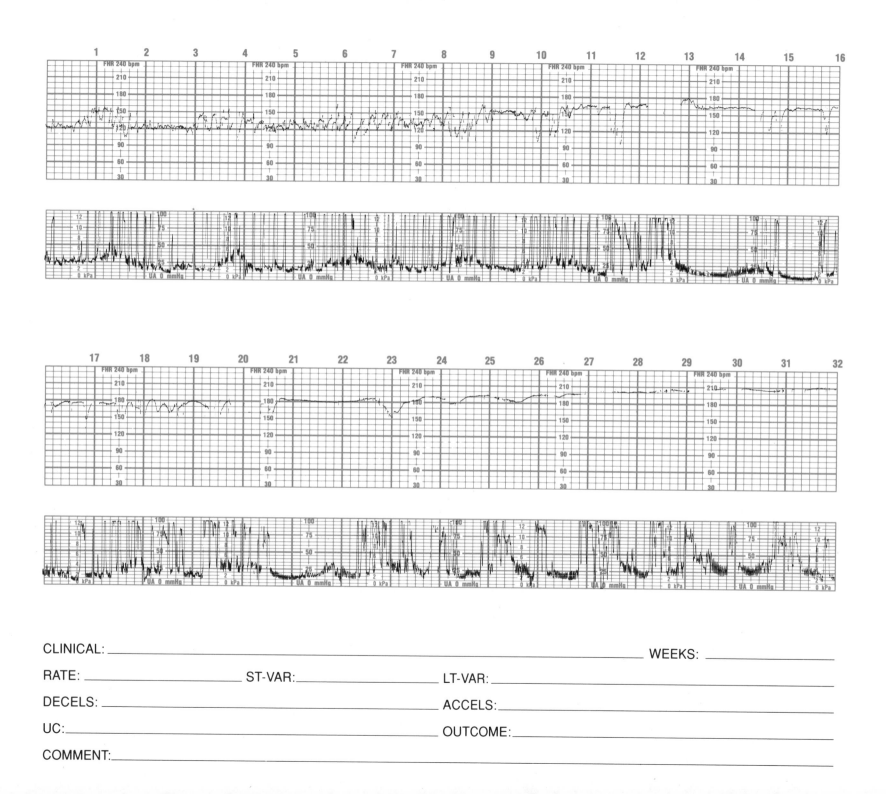

CLINICAL: _____ WEEKS: _____

RATE: _____ ST-VAR: _____ LT-VAR: _____

DECELS: _____ ACCELS: _____

UC: _____ OUTCOME: _____

COMMENT: _____

TRACING: 82

CLINICAL: Twins.

WEEKS: Preterm.

BASELINE RATE: 150

STV: Absent.

LTV: Absent.

DECELERATIONS: Variable.

ACCELERATIONS: None.

UC: None.

OUTCOME: Intracranial hemorrhage; neurologic handicap.

COMMENT: This tracing illustrates the evolution of the saw-tooth pattern as we have defined it. It must be emphasized that others use this term simply to describe increased variability—the saltatory pattern. This pattern was brought to my attention early one morning by the puzzled resident who asked, "Why did the infant do so poorly with all this variability?"

The tracing begins most ominously with several prolonged decelerations associated with absent baseline variability. Beginning just after 6M, the baseline is punctuated by abrupt, brief up-swings (about 10 bpm) followed by a more leisurely downslope. The duration of the entire deflection is less than 10 seconds. From that point on, the frequency of these excursions increases dramatically and predictably. Between 9M and 10M they appear with a frequency of 3–4/min. By 16M they appear with a frequency of 4–5/min. By 28M the frequency is simply too high to count. In addition, the amplitude decreases somewhat as the frequency increases. Because the excursions in this unusual case are well within the range of normal variability, one might look at a small segment of baseline (e.g., 10M–12M) and conclude that the variability was normal. But the overall progression of this baseline pattern should reveal how different this pattern is from normal baseline variability. Normal variability is random and unpredictable. The regularity and predictability of this pattern preclude their representing normal variability.

The commentary is continued on tracing 83.

REFERENCE

Freeman RK, Garite TJ, Nageotte MP: *Fetal Heart Rate Monitoring,* ed 2. Baltimore, Williams & Wilkins, 1991, pp 84–86.

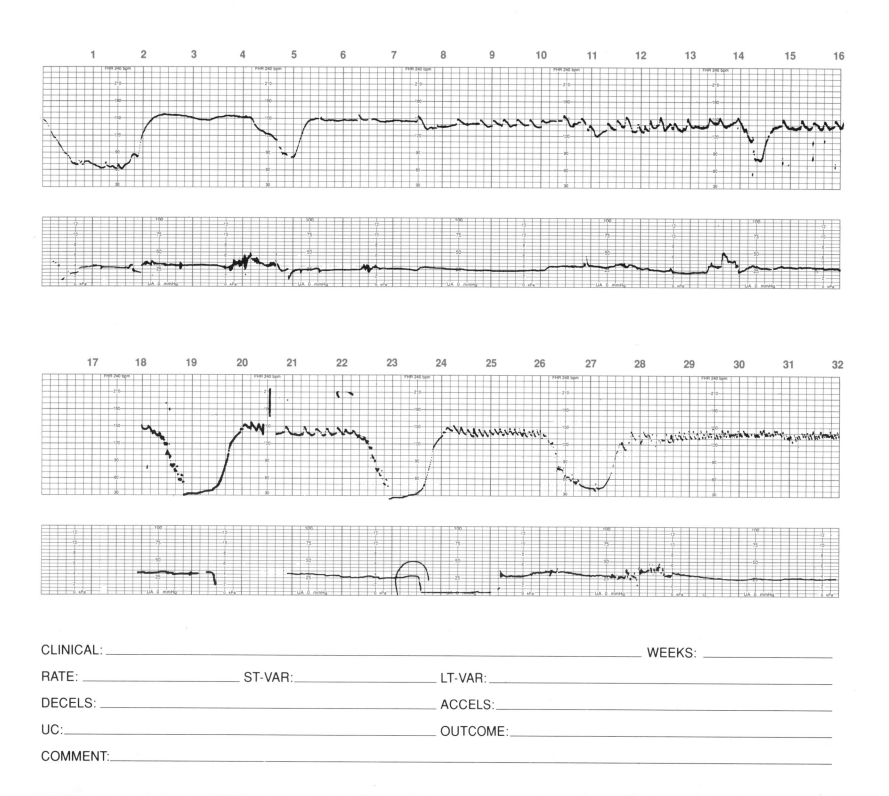

CLINICAL: _____ WEEKS: _____

RATE: _____ ST-VAR: _____ LT-VAR: _____

DECELS: _____ ACCELS: _____

UC: _____ OUTCOME: _____

COMMENT: _____

TRACING: 83

CLINICAL: Twins.

WEEKS: Preterm.

BASELINE RATE: 140

STV: Decreased.

LTV: Decreased.

DECELERATIONS: Variable.

ACCELERATIONS: None.

UC: Few.

OUTCOME: Intracranial hemorrhage (in utero); neurologic handicap.

COMMENT: These panels, a continuation of tracing 82, demonstrate the further progression of the sawtooth pattern. Note the continuing increase in the frequency and the concomitant decrease in the amplitude of the baseline oscillations that have replaced normal baseline variability.

The decelerations, variable and prolonged, could not be smoother or more rounded ("blunted"), but they have an inconstant relationship to the underlying contractions, which are not well recorded. Note that the decelerations themselves seem to be involved in the baseline oscillations, whereas the earlier decelerations, no more or no less severe, seem to be uninvolved by them.

It seems necessary to suggest that whatever injury had been visited on this fetus, it clearly antedated the appearance of the sawtooth pattern. The marked absence of variability, baseline tachycardia, and prolonged variable decelerations strongly suggest preexisting injury. Whether the sawtooth pattern represents the coup de grace, the final intracranial hemorrhage, or not, remains to be elucidated.

It should also be emphasized that this pattern would never have been seen or appreciated had external devices been used for the registration of the fetal heart rate. Reasonably, using an external device, the variability would probably have appeared diminished without evidence of these extraordinary oscillations in heart rate. Unfortunately, no comparison is available for this tracing. In all respects this tracing is quite ominous. Upon delivery, this infant, the first of preterm twins, was hopelessly depressed, although it survived, hopelessly handicapped. Neonatal examination revealed massive intracranial hemorrhage. The second twin had demonstrated a normal FHR tracing during labor, appeared normal at delivery, and survived intact.

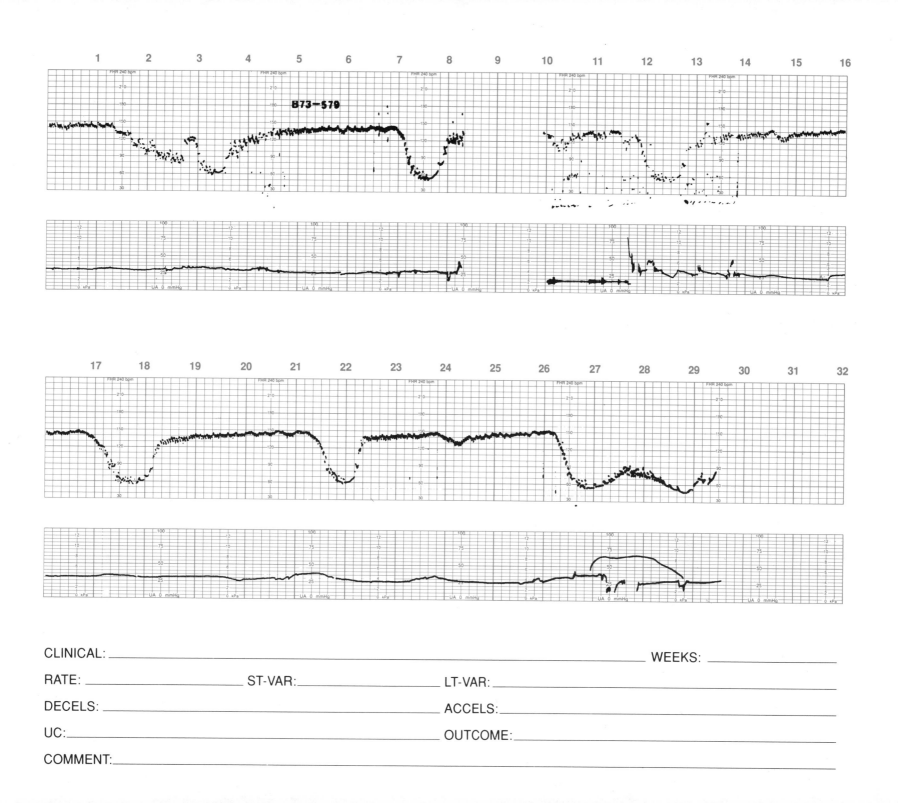

CLINICAL: _____ WEEKS: _____

RATE: _____ ST-VAR: _____ LT-VAR: _____

DECELS: _____ ACCELS: _____

UC: _____ OUTCOME: _____

COMMENT: _____

TRACING: 84

CLINICAL: Abdominal pain, bleeding, abruptio placentae.

WEEKS: 37

BASELINE RATE: 140–150

STV: Absent.

LTV: Absent.

DECELERATIONS: Variable.

ACCELERATIONS: Overshoot.

UC: Very frequent; polysystole.

OUTCOME: Apgar scores 0/1; profound neurological handicap.

COMMENT: This tracing is yet another example of using the FHR pattern to gain insight into preexisting neurologic injury in the fetus. In this instance contractions are coming very frequently in the second stage of labor, consistent with abruptio placentae. Each contraction is accompanied by maternal expulsive efforts. With each contraction the fetus responds with variable decelerations which return promptly to baseline. The baseline seems to fluctuate between absent variability and average variability. These designations, however, do not completely describe this unique tracing.

The baseline variability is extraordinarily flat except where it is punctuated by the sawtooth pattern (see below). The majority of the variable decelerations, irrespective of amplitude, are accompanied by small overshoot patterns. Although the baby spends most of its time decelerating, there is no real suggestion that the baseline heart rate is rising or that the fetal condition is deteriorating from the point of view of asphyxia.

There can be little question but that this tracing reflects significant neurologic abnormality. The sawtooth pattern seen between 5 and 6M, 12 and 13M, 15 and 16M, 18 and 19M, 21 and 22M, and in smaller snatches elsewhere, is a rare pattern usually associated with profound neurologic insult, intracranial hemorrhage, and death or profound disability.

As pointed out in the previous tracing, the major difficulty lies with the assumption that this sawtooth pattern represents "normal variability." To differentiate the sawtooth pattern from normal variability, one should focus on the regularity of the variability. Normal variability appears almost random, whereas in the case of the sawtooth pattern, even though the excursions may be in the normal range of variability, they are far too regular. The mechanism for the production of the sawtooth pattern is as yet unknown.

184

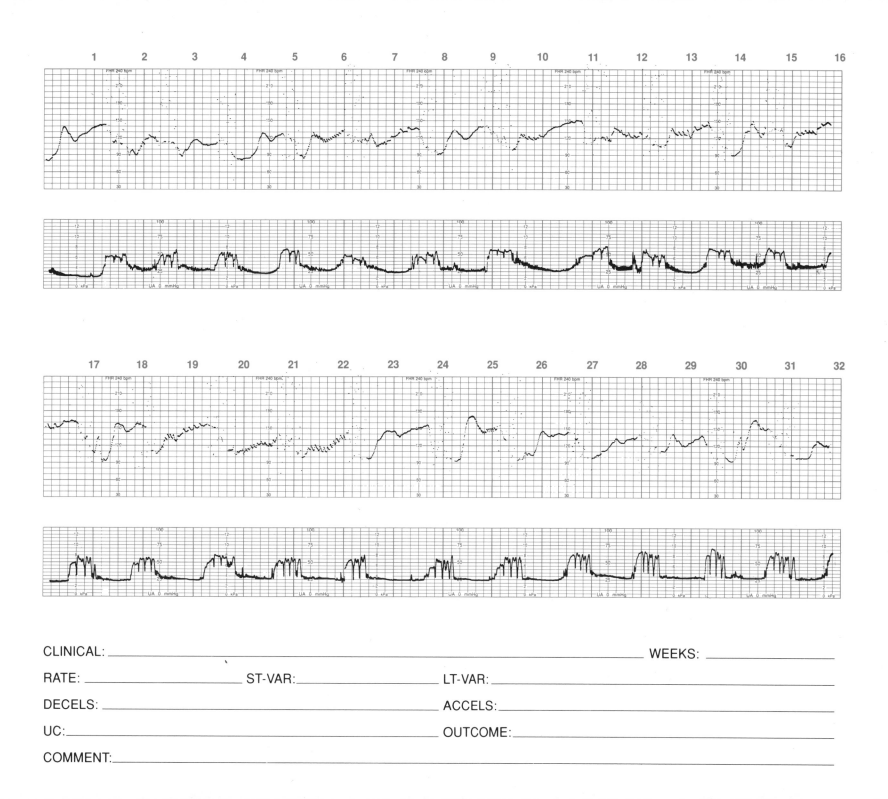

CLINICAL: _____   WEEKS: _____

RATE: _____ ST-VAR: _____   LT-VAR: _____

DECELS: _____   ACCELS: _____

UC: _____   OUTCOME: _____

COMMENT: _____

TRACING: 85

CLINICAL: Vaginal bleeding; labor.

WEEKS: 37

BASELINE RATE: 140

STV: Absent.

LTV: Absent.

DECELERATIONS: ?Late.

ACCELERATIONS: ?Uniform.

UC: Tachysystole.

OUTCOME: Forceps delivery; Apgar scores 1/1; neonatal death.

COMMENT: This is another tracing likely representing preexisting cerebral injury upon which is superimposed relatively acute asphyxia. In the *upper panel* there is an obvious lack of short-term variability and a stable baseline heart rate. The reader is left with the question of whether the periodic changes are accelerations with uterine contractions or late decelerations following the contractions. Because of the frequency of contractions, it is not possible to determine which is the case simply on the basis of the pattern. How shall we come to a conclusion? If these were late decelerations one would expect the decelerations to be consistent, and proportional in amplitude and duration to the amplitude and duration of the uterine contractions. But as the tracing progresses not only do the decelerations look less and less like late decelerations but they appear to disappear entirely. Looking at the *lower panel,* one would be hard-pressed to define a consistent pattern of late decelerations. In addition, there is no rise in baseline. If anything, during the *lower panel,* the FHR is falling.

Well, are they "accelerations" and do they represent a normal fetus? Not likely. These accelerations, which arise from absent variability, are associated with bizarre decelerations, and abrupt, angular changes in the heart rate do not comport with normal neurologic behavior. The lower half of the tracing, with its irregular undulating FHR pattern suggestive of the check-mark pattern and falling baseline rate, anticipates the hopeless condition of the neonate. This pattern not only suggests abnormal neurologic control over the heart rate but fetal shock as well. It does not represent normal long-term variability. Thus, whether the periodic changes in the *upper panel* are called "late decelerations" or "accelerations," there can be no optimism about the outcome of this fetus.

REFERENCE

Cruikshank DP: An unusual fetal heart rate pattern. *Am J Obstet Gynecol* 1978; 130:101.

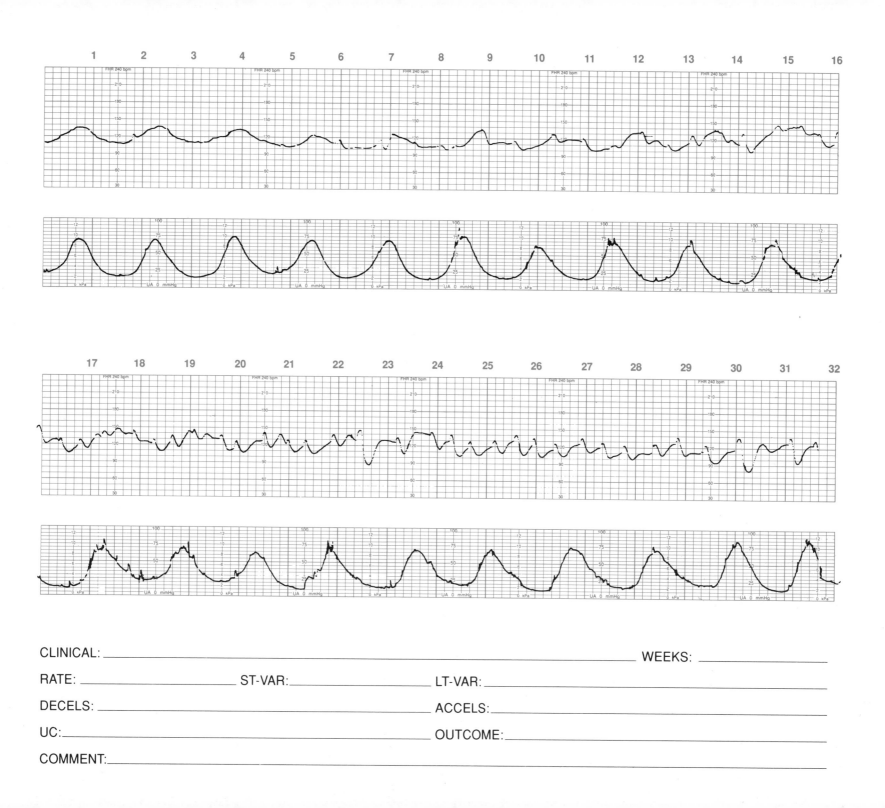

CLINICAL: _____ WEEKS: _____

RATE: _____ ST-VAR: _____ LT-VAR: _____

DECELS: _____ ACCELS: _____

UC: _____ OUTCOME: _____

COMMENT: _____

TRACING: 86

CLINICAL: Uneventful pregnancy.

WEEKS: 40

BASELINE RATE: 140–150

STV: Average.

LTV: Average.

DECELERATIONS: Early/variable; prolonged.

ACCELERATIONS: Sporadic.

UC: Irregular with occasional coupling; hypertonus; tachysystole.

OUTCOME: Midforceps rotation delivery; Apgar scores 2/8.

COMMENT: Initially the tracing reveals an unremarkable fetal heart rate pattern. The baseline is stable, variability is average, and brief, early or variable decelerations accompany most of the irregular contractions. Beginning at 22 minutes, just after the administration of epidural anesthesia with bupivacaine (Marcaine), the frequency of contractions increases dramatically with incomplete relaxation between the contractions (hypertonus). In response, the FHR falls to 90 bpm with minimal variability. This probably represents a nodal rhythm but no obvious or immediate danger to the fetus. But after a brief effort at recovery at 24M fails owing to the still frequent contractions, the FHR falls further, reaching 60 bpm. This secondary downturn in the heart rate represents a life-threatening situation for the fetus and the ultimate expression of "fetal distress." At the end of the tracing the patient is taken to the delivery room for operative delivery.

There is little doubt that this fetus is undergoing severe perinatal asphyxia and is at some risk of dying. These circumstances may also represent some potential for neurologic injury. It is not possible to determine injury from this tracing. In addition, this brief episode of asphyxia is unlikely, by itself, to cause injury. Having said this, it is important to bear in mind that mechanical factors are also operative here. The head is well down in the pelvis, and delivery will be assisted by midforceps operation. The role of mechanical effects on the causation of neurologic injury has not received adequate attention.

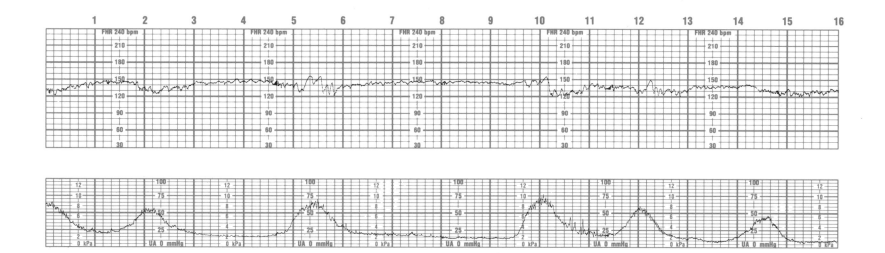

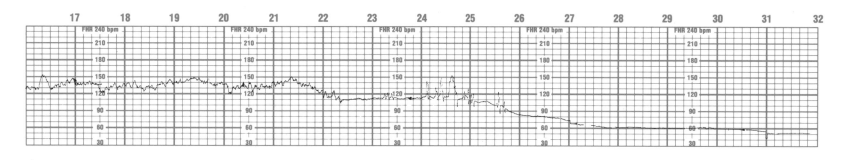

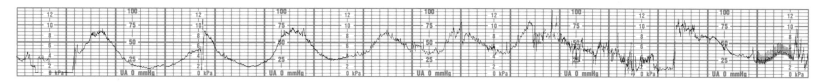

CLINICAL: _____ WEEKS: _____

RATE: _____ ST-VAR: _____ LT-VAR: _____

DECELS: _____ ACCELS: _____

UC: _____ OUTCOME: _____

COMMENT: _____

Index